W & H
Orthodontic Notes

ɔיK

25/5/03

Senior commissioning editor: Mary Seager
Editorial assistant: Caroline Savage
Production controller: Anthony Read
Desk editor: Claire Hutchins
Cover designer: Alan Studholme

W & H
Orthodontic Notes

Sixth edition

Edited and revised by

Malcolm L. Jones BDS (Wales) MSc (Lond) PhD (Wales) DOrth RCS (Eng)
FDS RCS (Edin)
Professor of Child Dental Health and Dean of the Dental School
University of Wales College of Medicine and
Consultant in Orthodontics

Richard G. Oliver BDS (Lond) MScD (Wales) PhD (Wales) LDS RCS (Eng)
FDS RCS (Edin)
Senior Lecturer in Orthodontics
University of Wales College of Medicine and
Consultant in Orthodontics

wright

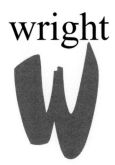

OXFORD AUCKLAND BOSTON JOHANNESBURG MELBOURNE NEW DELHI

Wright
An imprint of Butterworth-Heinemann
Linacre House, Jordan Hill, Oxford OX2 8DP
225 Wildwood Avenue, Woburn, MA 01801-2041
A division of Reed Educational and Professional Publishing Ltd

 A member of the Reed Elsevier plc group

First published 1960
Reprinted 1962, 1965
Second edition 1967
Reprinted 1972
Third edition 1976
Reprinted 1979
Fourth edition 1983
Reprinted 1985, 1990
Fifth edition 1994
Reprinted 1995, 1997, 1999
Sixth edition 2000

British Library Cataloguing in Publication Data
A catalogue record for this book is available from the British Library

Library of Congress Cataloguing in Publication Data
A catalogue record for this book is available from the Library of Congress

ISBN 0 7236 1065 7

Typeset by Keytec Typesetting Ltd, Bridport, Dorset
Printed and bound by MPG Books Ltd, Bodmin, Cornwall

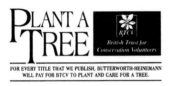

Contents

Contributors

Eli G. Absi DDS MSc PhD MSc Radiol
Senior Lecturer in Oral Radiology and
Consultant in Surgical Dentistry
University of Wales College of Medicine

Radiology in orthodontics – Chapter 19
Dento-alveolar surgery in relation to orthodontics – Chapter 20

Peter Durning BDS MSc DOrth MBA FDSRCS
Senior Lecturer and Consultant in Orthodontics,
University of Wales College of Medicine

Aetiology and management of the abnormally developing occlusion: interceptive orthodontics – Chapter 8

David Edmunds BDS MSc PhD FDSRCS (Eng)
Reader and Consultant in Restorative Dentistry,
University of Wales College of Medicine

The orthodontic–restorative interface – Chapter 24

Mike Hill BDS MDSc MSc MBA FDSRCS
Senior Lecturer in Oral and Maxillofacial Surgery;
Consultant Oral Surgeon,
University of Wales College of Medicine

Dento-alveolar surgery in relation to orthodontics – Chapter 20

Jeremy Knox BDS MSc PhD FDSRCS MOrth FDS (Orth)
Senior Lecturer in Orthodontics and
Consultant in Orthodontics
University of Wales College of Medicine

Retention and post-treatment relapse – Chapter 25

Stephen Richmond   BDS MScD PhD DOrth FDSRCS
Professor in Orthodontics and Dental Quality Assurance;
Consultant in Orthodontics
University of Wales College of Medicine

Orthodontic treatment need, complexity, outcome and cost-effectiveness –
Chapter 2

Adrian Sugar   BChD FDSRCS
Consultant in Maxillofacial Surgery,
The Welsh Centre for Burns, Plastic and Maxillofacial Surgery,
Morriston, Swansea, Wales, UK

The role of orthognathic surgery: planning and treatment – Chapter 22

Preface to the Sixth Edition

This book, first published in 1960, originally comprised the orthodontic notes taken from a series of lectures given to the undergraduate students at the Royal Dental Hospital, London, by Professor Walther.

In the preface to the first edition, Professor Walther stated that *Orthodontic Notes* were published in the hope that they might be of some use to other students. He intended that they should form the basis around which both the undergraduate and postgraduate student might read and develop a knowledge of the subject. Little was Professor Walther to know how successful this format was to become and how widely this small text was to be read: indeed, both of the current authors well remember referring to the second edition as undergraduates.

Following the early death of Professor Walther, Professor Houston was the natural successor to continue the updating and revision of the work, since he had been a Senior Lecturer at the Royal Dental Hospital and a contributor to the early editions.

After the untimely and tragic loss of Bill Houston we were approached by the publishers to take over the mantle of revising this book for a fifth edition in 1994. We have been gratified that the change in authors has had little effect on the popularity of this text. No doubt the format of producing a text of basic information, in the form of expanded notes, which is also competitively priced, is as popular with students now as it was in the 1960s!

Bill Houston's preface to the fourth edition is reprinted in full on the succeeding page to remind readers of the continuing purpose of this work. As we have approached the revision for a second time we have tried again to avoid the trap of radically changing the format. Therefore, we have followed the book's tradition of allowing the text to evolve whilst including new information, as appropriate, to reflect the changes in treatment approach and technique of recent years. Also, as in previous editions, we have aimed to keep this textbook simple, brief and basic, whilst avoiding detailed discussion wherever possible. In this edition, in response to constructive comments from the readership, we have included recommendations for further reading. We have deliberately avoided an exhaustive list of references, which are rarely referred to in any event! Readers will note that there are many changes, which largely consist of updating the text – a constant process. Some chapters have been extensively rewritten (see 'Growth of the facial skeleton'; 'Removable appliances'), others have seen a change in emphasis (see 'Orthodontic treatment need, complexity and cost-effectiveness'), whilst there are also completely new chapters (see 'Aetiology and management of the abnormally developing occlusion'; 'The orthodontic–restorative interface'; 'Retention and post-treatment relapse').

We hope that these notes continue to provide a straightforward theoretical base on which the postgraduate, undergraduate or general dental practitioner may build knowledge as they develop an interest in the speciality of orthodontics.

M.L.J and R.G.O.

Preface to the Fourth Edition

Since its first appearance in 1960, *Orthodontic Notes* has become a popular text with undergraduates. Although it has been reviewed extensively since that time, the intentions of Professor Walther have been followed: to present in a clear and concise fashion, the essentials of orthodontics required by undergraduate dental students and general dental practitioners. The brevity of presentation precludes detailed discussion of the many controversial topics in orthodontics. However, such debates are liable to be confusing rather than informative for the student who is being introduced to a subject. Thus a particular viewpoint is presented to hopefully provide a consistent and common sense framework of ideas. This should provide an adequate theoretical basis for the undergraduate student or general dental practitioner, and should form a sound foundation for the student who wishes to go further to specialize in orthodontics.

W.J.B.H.   1983

Acknowledgements

There are several people who have contributed to the production of this book without whose cheerful cooperation the task would have been arduous if not impossible.

In particular we would like to acknowledge the assistance of the Audiovisual Aids Department at the Dental School in Cardiff. This unit has reproduced the bulk of the illustrations, and we are grateful to Frank Hartles and Rodney Dollar for their help and expertise. Bryce Cumisky prepared the illustrations for Chapter 22 based on original artwork provided by Peter Evans, Chief Maxillo-facial Technologist at Morriston Hospital, Swansea.

We would also like to thank Mary Seager, Senior Commissioning Editor, Claire Hutchins, Desk Editor and the staff at Butterworth-Heinemann for their patient assistance.

We are pleased to have the opportunity here to acknowledge a debt of gratitude to Bill Houston and Norman Robertson, our respective teachers in the early stages of our orthodontic careers, for instilling into us an academic discipline of thought and deed, and leading by example. We are also grateful to the students, both undergraduate and postgraduate, whose searching questions keep us constantly thinking about what we are doing in orthodontics, and why.

Finally, as we did in the last edition, we would like to acknowledge the help and support of our wives. This hasn't just been moral support: Rhona Jones, with the benefit of a 'classical' education, has helped with grammar, punctuation and proofreading. Sheila Oliver, being dentally qualified (and therefore a potential reader of the book) has provided invaluable constructive comment.

Chapter 1

Introduction

Orthodontics has been defined as that branch of dental science concerned with the genetic variation, development and growth of facial form. It is also concerned with the manner in which these factors affect the occlusion of the teeth and the function of the associated organs.

Thus, whilst orthodontic techniques are concerned with the treatment of irregularities of the teeth, the study of orthodontics, as a whole, includes the growth, development and function of the total oro-facial complex. The aims of orthodontic treatment have been suggested to be the production of improved occlusal function by the correction of irregularities and, as a consequence, the creation of better dental health and improved aesthetics. It would be envisaged that such an improvement in personal appearance might later contribute to greater mental and physical well-being on the part of the individual patient. Whilst there might be some dispute as to whether all of these aims are routinely achievable in all patients, it is an important concept to grasp at the outset that no orthodontic treatment should ever cause harm to the patient. Such harm might occur by making the tooth arrangement or facial profile worse, or could involve leaving unsightly residual gaps after the inappropriate extraction of teeth. Where patient compliance is lacking during treatment, significant damage can also be done to teeth and gingivae. An example of this might be enamel decalcification (chalky marks) around a fixed appliance when the oral hygiene has not been properly managed. For these reasons a careful balance of benefit and risk must be made before commencing a course of orthodontic treatment.

Also it is important that each treatment, and thus each appliance approach, should be matched to the individual patient. Similarly, the appropriate level of professional skill should also be matched to the presenting problem. This will mean that whilst some patients may be treated by simple means in the general dental practice environment, many others will require referral to a specialist practitioner with training in more advanced techniques.

The general dental practitioner (GDP) attends to the dental well-being of the patient. This includes both the monitoring and management of the developing occlusion. They should have sufficient orthodontic knowledge to enable them to know when they might intervene to improve tooth arrangement but also when it is best to refer for either an expert opinion or a more complex treatment. Thus the GDP has the very important role of 'gatekeeper' to orthodontic care.

Ideal occlusion is a hypothetical concept based on the anatomy of the teeth. It is rarely, if ever, found in nature. However, it provides a standard by which all other occlusions may be judged. Normal occlusion (Figure 1.1) is commonly described as 'An occlusion within the accepted deviation of the ideal'. This vague definition means that there are no clear limits to the range of normal occlusion. However, in general, minor variations in the alignment of the teeth which are not of aesthetic or functional importance might be considered as being consistent with a normal occlusion. Edward Angle, who is credited with the modern development of orthodontics as a speciality, provided the first clear definition of the normal occlusion. He related it to the arrangement of the occlusal contact of the first permanent molars, the mesial buccal cusp of the maxillary first permanent molar occluding with the mid-buccal groove of the opposing mandibular first permanent molar. He suggested that if such a relationship existed and the teeth were arranged in a smoothly curving line of occlusion then a normal occlusion would be the result.

Malocclusion is an irregularity in the occlusion beyond the accepted range of normal. The fact that an individual has a malocclusion is not in itself a justification for treatment. Only if it is possible to say with certainty that the patient will benefit aesthetically or functionally, and only if they are suitable and willing to undergo treatment should orthodontic intervention be considered. In other words, it is not sufficient for there to be a professional perception of need – it should also be matched by a demand for treatment by the patient in order to 'trigger' the commencement of a plan to correct the malocclusion.

Orthodontics – the beginnings

Edward Angle has been called the 'father of modern orthodontics'. He published the first attempts at defining the problem through the development of a classification system (1890), still in current use, and suggested an 'ideal' treatment aim. Further, he developed treatment systems to achieve those aims including the first 'edgewise' fixed appliance (1928) – a system which still provides the basis of the majority of orthodontic appliances being used world-

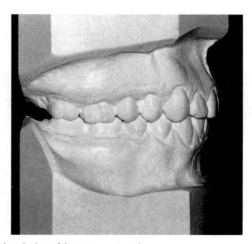

Figure 1.1 Normal occlusion of the permanent teeth

wide at the start of the twenty-first century. He also established the first postgraduate training school in the USA.

However, it is important to be aware that the ideas and concepts behind orthodontic treatment have been around for a very much longer period of time. Apparently the Etruscans were using crude devices as early as the eighth century BC in an attempt to move displaced teeth. The first published reference to applying a load to move a tooth is to be found in *De medicina*, an encyclopedia of medicine produced by Aulus Celsus, a famous Roman physician who flourished early in the first century AD. Curiously, it would appear that this text was still being used in the eighteenth century, being translated into English as late as 1756!

The scope and aims of orthodontic treatment

These might be best summarized as follows:

1. The improvement of facial and dental aesthetics.
2. The alignment of the teeth to eliminate stagnation areas.
3. The elimination of premature contacts which give rise to mandibular displacements and may contribute to later muscle or joint pain.
4. The elimination of traumatic irregularities of the teeth (Figure 1.2).
5. The alignment of prominent teeth which are liable to be damaged.
6. The alignment of irregular teeth prior to bridgework, crowns or partial dentures.
7. The alignment of periodontally involved teeth prior to splinting.
8. The alignment and planned positioning of teeth in the jaws prior to orthognathic surgery.
9. To assist the eruption and alignment of displaced teeth.

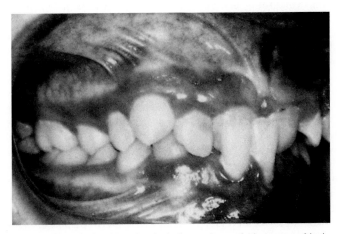

Figure 1.2 A traumatic occlusion. Note the gingival recession on the lower central incisors

Orthodontic treatment options

There are seven basic treatment approaches to the management and correction of malocclusion.

1. **No treatment.** This involves the acceptance of mild irregularity on the principle that limited crowding will often be far better than any residual post-treatment extraction space or prolonged fixed appliance treatment to close these spaces. Limited resources should be concentrated on patients with more severe malocclusions.
2. **Extraction only.** To be considered only where the degree and position of crowding are favourable, as are the local tooth angulations. Extraction of teeth will allow spontaneous movement and may provide an acceptable result in a limited number of cases. Such an approach is most appropriate when planned deciduous tooth extraction is considered as part of a treatment in the mixed dentition (see Chapter 8).
3. **Removable appliance treatment.** Where tooth position, inclination and angulations are favourable, a removable appliance may correct a malocclusion by simple tipping movements about the apical third of the root (see Chapter 16). Removable appliances are most efficient and are best tolerated in the upper dental arch.
4. **Single arch fixed appliances.** These may be used where there are limited treatment aims, usually involving corrections of either rotations or angulations of teeth. They may, on occasion, be used in the lower arch for the purposes of alignment or for space closure where bodily movement is necessary. In this situation it may, occasionally, be used in conjunction with an upper removable appliance.
5. **Full upper and lower arch fixed appliances.** These appliances, usually, are attached to all erupted maxillary and mandibular teeth and allow full correction of all teeth in three planes of space (see Chapter 17).
6. **Functional (including orthopaedic) appliances.** Functional appliances are specialized removable appliances which consist of upper and lower segments, which may be fixed together, or close together, such as to hold the mandibular dental arch in a postured position. They are most appropriately employed in those patients with retrusive mandibular teeth and jaw. These appliances appear to be most effective in patients where there is current active growth (see Chapter 18). Orthopaedic appliances may be either removable or fixed, and are used to specifically effect a movement of the facial bones. An example might be rapid maxillary expansion (RME), which usually forms part of an appliance used to split the mid-palatal suture and thus expand the maxilla. Some designs of functional appliance may also have an orthopaedic role and vice versa.
7. **Orthognathic surgery.** This is a complex treatment approach involving a combination of both fixed appliances and surgery to the jaws. By such means large discrepancies of the jaws may be corrected in suitable patients when growth has largely ceased (see Chapter 22). Careful planning, together with the timing of surgery demand early, and expert, interspeciality appraisal.

The timing of orthodontic treatment

The deciduous dentition

Treatment at this stage is hardly ever indicated. Examples of possible exceptions are where a malpositioned tooth may give rise to marked mandibular displacement, or where a supernumerary tooth is creating a localized problem. However, it is important to identify and make an early referral for those patients where significant jaw discrepancy or facial asymmetry are apparent during these early stages of growth.

The early mixed dentition

The planned extraction of extensively carious first permanent molars, balancing extractions of deciduous teeth, and serial extractions may be undertaken during this stage (see Chapters 8 and 16). Space maintainers may be fitted and simple orthodontic treatment to correct an instanding incisor or alternatively to eliminate a mandibular displacement may be indicated (see Chapters 9 and 16). Only treatment which can be completed rapidly and which will be stable should be attempted. Prolonged appliance wear at this stage is to be avoided and is unlikely, in any event, to be longer than between three and six months. The types of treatment that are employed in the early mixed dentition are intended to either eliminate or, at a minimum, reduce the severity of a developing malocclusion. A term often applied to this type of occlusal management is 'interceptive orthodontics'. It is at this time that such measures are most often employed (see Chapter 8).

The late mixed and early permanent dentition

At this stage, the greater part of orthodontic treatment is carried out. Most of the permanent teeth have erupted and there is little further growth in arch width, thus crowding can be reliably estimated. In the majority of children the jaw relationship changes only to a limited extent after the age of ten years (Chapter 2) and so it is possible to plan and carry out orthodontic treatment with the confidence that major growth changes are not likely to affect the treatment adversely. It is at this stage that most definitive active treatment to correct malocclusion will be performed, and it has been suggested that children in this age group are often more willing to wear appliances than are older adolescents and adults.

The late permanent dentition

It is important to recognize that orthodontic treatment may be undertaken at almost any age. In North America and Western Europe an increasing number of treatments are being undertaken for the adult patient. However, treatment planning and mechanics will usually require modification from that which is appropriate in the growing child (Chapter 21).

Whatever the age of the patient, when treatment is being considered, a careful assessment of need, taking into account the balance of benefit and cost (which could include emotional, clinical and financial cost), must be made in partnership with the patient and, where appropriate, with the parents. Consideration must be given to the process of informed consent. A factor in this process is to have available appropriate information on the effectiveness of any treatment approaches being considered, and for the clinician to have the ability to adequately communicate that information to the patient.

The assessment of treatment need and the decision to treat is explored in more detail in the next chapter.

Further reading

Angle, E.H. (1900). *Treatment of Malocclusion of the Teeth and Fractures of the Maxillae, Angle's System*. Philadelphia: S.S. White Dental Co.

Angle, E.H. (1928). The latest and best in orthodontic mechanisms. *Dental Cosmos*, **70**, 1143–58.

Asbell, M.B. (1990). A brief history of orthodontics. *American Journal of Orthodontics and Dentofacial Orthopedics*, **97**, 206–13.

Corrucini, R.S. and Pacciani, E. (1989). 'Orthodontistry' and dental occlusion in the Etruscans. *Angle Orthodontist*, **59**, 61–4.

Chapter 2

Orthodontic treatment need, complexity, outcome and cost-effectiveness

Need and demand for treatment

Health care professionals are often asked to demonstrate that orthodontic services are appropriately allocated and that if treatment has been undertaken that the patients have benefited from the intervention.

When assessing orthodontic treatment need it is important to establish 'cause and effect'. As an example, the risk of fractured incisors in an 8–10-year-old is substantially increased when the overjet is greater than 6 mm. It is important to build an 'evidence-based system' to determine which deviant occlusal traits, either in isolation or in combination, pose a threat to the longevity of the dentition and surrounding structures. The adverse effects of a malocclusion should also be considered within the broader concept of the 'quality of life'. This could be considered in terms of the individual's social-psychological development, long-term ambitions and potential achievement.

Malocclusion is a continuum, ranging from an ideal occlusion to considerable deviations from normal. Assessing 'cut-off' levels in deciding who might benefit from treatment and those that might not, can be difficult. The severity of the malocclusion, the appliance type to be employed, the skill of the operator and the potential cooperation of the patient all have to be taken into account. Whilst making these types of decision it is important to remember that the main aim of orthodontic care is to eliminate or reduce the adverse effects that may result from any malocclusion.

Demand for orthodontic treatment results from an individual's desire to seek treatment due to a perceived (usually observed) problem with the dentition and/ or surrounding structures. Figure 2.1 illustrates the interaction of professional need (e.g. assessed by the dentist) with the individual's demand for orthodontic treatment.

If the professional indicates a need for treatment and the individual desires treatment then the treatment can progress in an environment where there are appropriate resources (e.g. appropriately trained staff, facilities and materials). However, if the resources are either not available or insufficient, an unmet treatment need and demand will result. If the professional determines an objective need in the individual but the individual does not wish to have treatment then this is termed a 'potential professional objective need'. These individuals may or may not wish to proceed with treatment at a later date. In a situation where the individual perceives a problem but there is no significant

Need and Demand
for Orthodontic Treatment

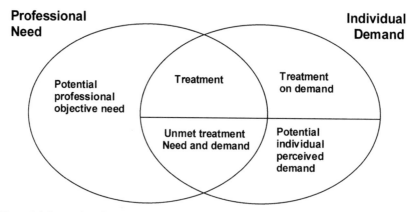

Professional Need

Individual Demand

Potential professional objective need

Treatment

Treatment on demand

Unmet treatment Need and demand

Potential individual perceived demand

Figure 2.1 Interaction of treatment need (as assessed by dentist) with patient's demand for orthodontic treatment

objective need assessment the practitioner may still choose to enter treatment to satisfy that demand. However, if the practitioner refuses treatment there will be a 'potential individual perceived demand' for orthodontic care.

A collection of surveys has been compiled in which professional need has been identified with various populations around the world (Table 2.1).

The professionally determined need varies widely and depends on the criteria used, which could include: age, gender, type of population studied and the 'cut-off' levels for severity of malocclusion. The data would suggest that the professionally determined need appears to range from 27.5 to 76.7%. Fewer studies have identified the demand for treatment by a population but this would appear to range from 2 to 47%.

The need and demand for orthodontic care fluctuates through an individual's life due to different 'life cycle events' including change in wealth and social conditions (personal, national and international). Need and demand are also influenced by the dental development, facial growth, social awareness and culture, as well as dentist interventions due to dental decay and loss of teeth.

Indices to measure orthodontic treatment need

Numerous occlusal indices have been developed to categorize individuals according to urgency and need for treatment. The aims of these indices are to:

- record treatment need in a population and assign priority to types of malocclusions
- record health gain resulting from treatment
- apportion resources, including finance, health care workers and facilities.

The Index of Orthodontic Treatment Need (IOTN) is one of the best known and most extensively validated of these indices. It attempts to find and rank

Table 2.1 International studies for treatment need and demand

	Index	Type of sample	Age group	% Need	% Demand
Argentina	WHO-FDI	1554	12–13	Amerindian 18 Caucasian 28	
Denmark	Björk et al.	Representative 531	9–10	70	
England and Wales	IOTN	Representative 10, 291	9–15	9 years 31 5–15 years 15–33 11–12 years 27.5	12 years 16
Finland	Björk et al.	Representative 100 boys 100 girls	7.7	23.5 need 34.5 observation	
Japan	Dental Aesthetic Index	409	15–18	22 Crowding 40	
Kenya	Norwegian Orthodontic Treatment Index (NOTI)	91	13–15	29	33
Norway	Norwegian Orthodontic Treatment Index (NOTI)	93	11	65	47
The Netherlands	Own	Representative	15–74	15 years 35–39 62.4	15–19 years 23.5
Saudi Arabia	Björk et al.	500 males	14	Male 35 Female 40	Male 8 Female 11
Sweden	Björk et al.	920	>20	Minor 22 Definite 25 Severe 8 Very severe 5	
Turkey	Treatment Priority Index		6–10		
USA	Own	3696 Representative		Females 42 Males 44 White 46 Black 36	Females 9.5 Males 6.8 White 12 Black 1 High social class 12 Low social class 2
Zambia	Summer's Occlusal Index	601	9–12	17	

malocclusions in terms of the significance of various occlusal traits for an individual's dental health and perceived aesthetic impairment. The intention is to identify those individuals who would receive the greatest benefit from orthodontic treatment. The Index incorporates an Aesthetic Component and Dental Health Component. The Aesthetic Component consists of 10 photographs showing different levels of dental attractiveness. Individual cases can be identified and ranked according to this scale (Figure 2.2). The Dental Health Component ranks deviant occlusal traits based on available evidence (Figure 2.3). The more severe the deviant occlusal trait, the greater the need for orthodontic treatment. When this index is applied to a typical population of 11–12-year-old children approximately one-third fall into grades 4 and 5 (most need), another third fall into grade 3 and a further third occupy grades 1 and 2 (least need).

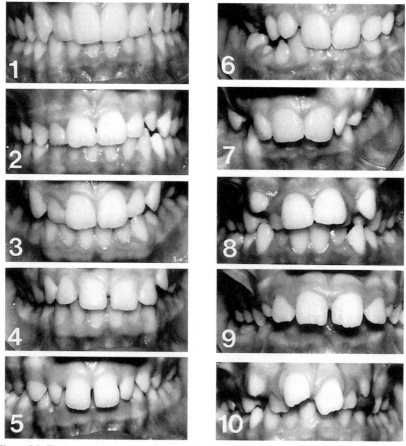

Figure 2.2 The Aesthetic Component of the Index of Orthodontic Treatment Need: the severity of the appearance of the malocclusion is matched to the nearest example and the score (1–10) is recorded

THE DENTAL HEALTH COMPONENT
OF THE INDEX OF ORTHODONTIC TREATMENT NEED (IOTN)

GRADE 5 (Need treatment)

5.i Impeded eruption of teeth (except for third molars) due to crowding, displacement, the presence of supernumerary teeth, retained deciduous teeth and any pathological cause.

5.h Extensive hypodontia with restorative implications (more than 1 tooth missing in any quadrant) requiring pre-restorative orthodontics.

5.a Increased overjet greater than 9mm.

5.m Reverse overjet greater than 3.5mm with reported masticatory and speech difficulties.

5.p Defects of cleft lip and palate and other craniofacial anomalies.

5.s Submerged deciduous teeth.

GRADE 3 (Borderline need)

3.a Increased overjet greater than 3.5mm but less than or equal to 6mm with incompetent lips.

3.b Reverse overjet greater than 1mm but less than or equal to 3.5mm.

3.c Anterior or posterior crossbites with greater than 1mm but less than or equal to 2mm discrepancy between retruded contact position and intercuspal position.

3.d Contact point displacements greater than 2mm but less than or equal to 4mm.

3.e Lateral or anterior open bite greater than 2mm but less than or equal to 4mm.

3.f Deep overbite complete on gingival or palatal tissues but no trauma.

GRADE 4 (Need treatment)

4.h Less extensive hypodontia requiring pre-restorative orthodontics or orthodontic space closure to obviate the need for a prosthesis.

4.a Increased overjet greater than 6mm but less than or equal to 9mm.

4.b Reverse overjet greater than 3.5mm with no masticatory or speech difficulties.

4.m Reverse overjet greater than 1mm but less than 3.5mm with recorded masticatory and speech difficulties.

4.c Anterior or posterior crossbites with greater than 2mm discrepancy between retruded contact position and intercuspal position.

4.l Posterior lingual crossbite with no functional occlusal contact in one or both buccal segments.

4.d Severe contact point displacements greater than 4mm.

4.e Extreme lateral or anterior open bites greater than 4mm.

4.f Increased and complete overbite with gingival or palatal trauma.

4.t Partially erupted teeth, tipped and impacted against adjacent teeth.

4.x Presence of supernumerary teeth.

GRADE 2 (Little)

2.a Increased overjet greater than 3.5mm but less than or equal to 6mm with competent lips.

2.b Reverse overjet greater than 0mm but less than or equal to 1mm.

2.c Anterior or posterior crossbite with less than or equal to 1mm discrepancy between retruded contact position and intercuspal position.

2.d Contact point displacements greater than 1mm but less than or equal to 2mm.

2.e Anterior or posterior openbite greater than 1mm but less than or equal to 2mm.

2.f Increased overbite greater than or equal to 3.5mm without gingival contact.

2.g Pre-normal or post-normal occlusions with no other anomalies (includes up to half a unit discrepancy).

GRADE 1 (None)

1. Extremely minor malocclusions including contact point displacements less than 1mm.

Figure 2.3 The Dental Health Component of the Index of Orthodontic Treatment Need

Indices to record treatment standards

These indices compare pre- and post-treatment records to record the outcome of orthodontic care. One index that has been developed to perform this task is called the PAR Index (Peer Assessment Rating). The PAR Index records the technical quality of care, standard of treatment and the degree of improvement as a result of any intervention. This index is useful in determining the efficiency and effectiveness of orthodontic care, allowing a clinician to self-assess (audit) their results whilst also being applicable to the wider context of comparison of health care delivery systems both nationally and internationally. Such an index may also be applied in the assessment of treatment modalities. For example, malocclusions in England and Wales are generally reduced by an average of over 70% if upper and lower fixed appliances are employed, whilst routine use of upper removable appliances will usually achieve less than 50% improvement.

Indices to record treatment complexity

Complexity may be defined as 'something which is complicated or intricate'. An alternative definition of orthodontic treatment complexity could be 'the recognition and management of problems during the treatment process to optimize the result'. This definition implies that complexity only becomes an important factor during the treatment process. The difficulty lies in predicting what case is going to be difficult prior to treatment. Not surprisingly, a retrospective assessment of the complexity is much easier to make and could be based on such factors as: increased number of appointments, increased length of appointments, the age of the patient or initial severity of the malocclusion (as defined by the PAR score).

However, systems are being developed to predict a treatment's complexity. One such index being developed for international use is the Index of Complexity, Outcome and Need (ICON). So far, it appears to have promise in fulfilling its aim of objectively assessing complexity, as well as outcome and need. This index has obvious advantages in trying to combine three indices into just one. The ICON has five basic components which combine aspects of the IOTN and PAR index. These are the 'Aesthetic Component', the assessment of upper arch crowding/spacing, an assessment of presence/absence of crossbite, a measure of the degree of overbite/open bite, and a check of the 'fit' of the buccal occlusion.

The use of the occlusal indices (IOTN, ICON and PAR) is illustrated in Figure 2.4.

Risk–benefit assessment

Risk is defined as the probability that a particular adverse event will occur during a stated period of time. The adverse event is an occurrence that produces harm. Benefit is the gain to the patient. Expected benefit incorporates the probability of achieving the intended health gain.

The risks of orthodontic treatment have been well documented and might include:

- root resorption
- enamel decalcification
- gingival swelling, gingivitis
- trauma from attachments – ulceration
- allergies from nickel and latex
- incomplete treatment
- relapse
- loss of tooth vitality

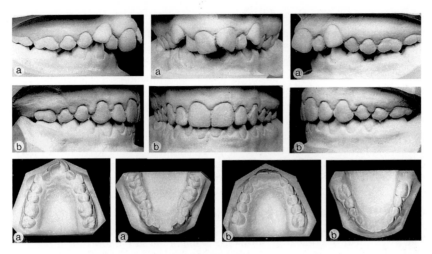

Figure 2.4 The application of occlusal indices IOTN PAR and ICON

	Index of Orthodontic Treatment Need (IOTN)			
	Aesthetic Component (AC)	Dental Health Component (DHC)	Peer Assessment Rating (PAR)	Index of Complexity, Outcome and Need (ICON)
Pre-treatment (a)	9	5.a	40	98
Post-treatment (b)	2	2.g	2	20

- bacteraemia from placement of bands
- patient not satisfied with treatment result.

However, the perceived benefits from orthodontic treatment are more difficult to define due to lack of strong scientific evidence to support the links between deviant malocclusions and disease. The benefits may include:

- improving psychological well-being
- improving self-esteem and popularity
- improving dental and facial attractiveness
- improving function (mastication and speech)
- reducing the risk of trauma to incisors where there is an increased overjet
- reducing the pathological migration of teeth in later life
- aligned teeth may facilitate easier tooth cleaning
- improving facial symmetry
- improving periodontal support or reducing the continued loss or rate of loss of periodontal support
- reducing the problems associated with impacted and missing teeth
- support of multidisciplinary approaches with other dental specialities to produce optimum facial and dental attractiveness in addition to function.

Risk evaluation is a complex process of determining the significance of possible adverse events. Therefore it includes the study of risk perception and the 'trade-off' between perceived risks and perceived benefits. It is the responsibility of the clinician to notify the patient of the likelihood of possible adverse events in the context of the probable outcome of treatment with minor malocclusions the risks of treatment may outweigh the perceived benefits. In addition, certain types of malocclusion are associated with poorer outcomes. For example, open bites tend to be successfully treated in only 60% of cases. Surgical correction of Class III malocclusions can result in a relapse, on average, of 25% whilst relapse in surgically corrected Class II malocclusions can be greater than 30%. In association with surgical procedures other risks might include death due to an adverse reaction to an anaesthetic or more commonly (and less drastic) nerve damage resulting in lip paraesthesia.

Cost-effectiveness of orthodontic care

The assessment of clinical performance is important at the individual, practice, institutional and national level. It is a challenge not only to deliver high standards of care but also to deliver this care at the lowest unit cost. An index such as the PAR Index facilitates the assessment of cost-effectiveness. The estimated costs of delivering orthodontic care are illustrated in (Table 2.2). It is important to assess the overall cost in terms of reduction in unit malocclusion and cost per visit. Interestingly, the cost per unit reduction of malocclusion is similar to cost per visit for orthodontic care in Norway and in the community dental service in the UK. In contrast, the cost per visit for specialists and non-specialists is much higher than cost per unit reduction. This is related to the duration of treatment since the treatment time is much reduced with only a marginal increase in the finish PAR score. In other words the biggest, most worthwhile, PAR reductions occur early in the treatment cycle.

Treatment duration is very variable from country to country and, to some extent, depends on the type of service in which it is delivered and also the local health care and remuneration system. An average treatment duration of 36 months in The Netherlands is high compared to 16 and 17 months in the UK, but curiously leads to no difference in the finished result as measured by the PAR score. To some extent, duration of treatment is influenced by the severity of the malocclusion, level of training, experience of the clinician, type of monitoring techniques employed during treatment, aspirations of the clinician, method of remuneration, and the health care system. The average number (per

Table 2.2 Examples of cost-effectiveness in different countries and settings

Cost per unit reduction in PAR score (∈)	Cost per visit (∈)	Duration of treatment (months)	Cost (∈, euro)	Finish PAR score	Setting where the study was undertaken
45	43	24	869	4	Specialist practice (Norway)
30	33	25	620	6	Community clinics (UK)
28	47	17	659	7	Specialist orthodontist (UK)
35	51	16	659	8	Non-specialist orthodontists (UK)
–	–	36	–	8	Hospital care (The Netherlands)
–	–	30	–	6	Extraction cases (hospital, USA)
–	–	26	–	6	Non-extraction cases (hospital, USA)

orthodontist) of completed orthodontic cases per year in England and Wales is 300. However, in the international context, the case load is determined by many factors, including: the speed of the operator; the use of auxiliaries; the type of national remuneration system; the level of remuneration; and the income that is desired, on average, by the orthodontist. Generally, there is a tendency for lower levels of remuneration to be associated with higher caseloads.

Conclusion

The use of occlusal indices ensures uniform interpretation and application of criteria. It is important before applying indices to confirm that they are valid (i.e. that they measure what they purport to measure) and reliable (i.e. the ability of the same examiner and different examiners to achieve the same score). There is a necessity to improve diagnostic criteria and develop a common approach to assessing treatment need and treatment outcome (based on available evidence). Patients who enter into a treatment should be treated with the most effective appliances by those practitioners most competent to perform treatment to a high standard. In addition to the ethical need for effective orthodontic treatment, consideration should also be given to delivering orthodontic care at a reasonable cost over an optimal period of time.

Further reading

Brook, P.H. and Shaw, W.C. (1989). The development of an index of orthodontic treatment priority. *European Journal of Orthodontics*, **11**, 309–20.

Heikinheimo, K. (1978). Need of orthodontic treatment in 7-year-old Finnish children. *Community Dental and Oral Epidemiology*, **6**, 129–34.

Helm, S., Kreiborg, S., Barlebo, J. *et al.* (1975). Estimates of orthodontic treatment need in Danish schoolchildren. *Community Dental and Oral Epidemiology*, **3**, 136–42.

Hill, P.A. (1992). The prevalence and severity of malocclusion and the need for orthodontic treatment in 9, 12, and 15-year-old Glasgow schoolchildren. *British Journal of Orthodontics*, **19**, 87–96.

Holman, J.K., Hans, M.G., Nelson, S. *et al.* (1998). An assessment of extraction versus nonextraction orthodontic treatment using the peer assessment rating (PAR) index. *Angle Orthodontist*, **68**, 527–34.

Holmes, A. (1992). The subjective need and demand for orthodontic treatment. *British Journal of Orthodontics*, **19**, 287–97.

Prahl-Andersen, B. (1978). The need for orthodontic treatment. *Angle Orthodontist*, **48**, 1–9.

Proffit, W.R., Fields, H.W., Moray, L.J. *et al.* (1998). Prevalence of malocclusion and orthodontic treatment need in the United States: estimates from the NHANES III survey. *International Journal of Adult Orthodontics and Orthognathic Surgery*, **13**, 97–106.

Richmond, S. (2000). The need for cost-effectiveness. *Journal of Orthodontics*, **27**, 275–6.

Richmond, S. and Andrews, M. (1993). Orthodontic treatment standards in Norway. *European Journal of Orthodontics*, **15**, 7–15.

Salonen, L., Mohlin, B., Gotzlinger, B. *et al.* (1992). Need and demand for orthodontic treatment in an adult Swedish population. *European Journal of Orthodontics*, **14**, 359–68.

Wheeler, T.T., McGorray, S.P., Yurkiewicz, L. *et al.* (1994). Orthodontic treatment demand and need in third and fourth grade schoolchildren. *American Journal of Orthodontics and Dentofacial Orthopedics*, **106**, 22–33.

Chapter 3

Growth of the facial skeleton

Growth and development

Why should a dentist or orthodontist be interested in growth and development?

1. Knowledge of general and facial growth provides a background to the understanding of the aetiology and development of malocclusion. Such an understanding is, in turn, an important part of the diagnosis and treatment planning process.
2. As observers, at regular intervals, of the growing child all dentists should be able to identify abnormal or unusual patterns of skeletal growth and refer as appropriate.
3. More particularly, the dentist should be able to identify abnormal occlusal development at an early stage in order to undertake suitable interceptive orthodontic treatment where appropriate. Occlusal development is obviously closely linked to facial growth and development.
4. Inopportune and/or poorly timed extractions performed by the dentist during growth may have unfortunate consequences on the developing occlusion.
5. Many malocclusions are, at least in part, due to skeletal discrepancies between the jaws (maxilla and mandible). Such discrepancies are usually due to differences in the comparative growth of the jaws. More severe malocclusions may be related to more distant skeletal discrepancies within the cranial base. Correctly identifying these growth features may be important in deciding upon a diagnosis and formulating a treatment plan.
6. Orthodontic treatment may make use of growth spurts and other trends. The timing of treatment in relation to these may be important. Tooth movement is more rapid the greater the growth activity. For both these reasons an understanding of the kinetics of facial growth is necessary.
7. Most orthodontic treatments are performed in the actively growing child or adolescent. Some are dependent on favourable growth and these treatments may have an effect on the hard and soft tissues of the area.
8. In some treatments, for example where surgery is being considered, it is important to be able to identify when the majority of facial growth has been completed.
9. Growth effects can have long-term effects on the stability of the occlusion after treatment. This needs to be considered when a retention regime is planned.

General growth and development

The contrast between prenatal and postnatal growth

One may define growth as an increase in size, whilst development is the progress towards maturity; each process is obviously intertwined with the other, but it is important to recognize that there is some difference between the two processes. It is also important to appreciate the speed and complexity of cell multiplication and differentiation, particularly during the prenatal stage of growth and development. During this period the height increase is 5000-fold. In contrast, postnatally it is three-fold. Similarly the weight increase from ovum to birth is 6.5 billion-fold and from birth to adulthood is ten-fold.

During the first few months of life after birth, growth is at its postnatal peak. For example, by the end of the fourth month the birth weight has usually doubled; if growth continued at this rate a man would be 1000 lbs (450 kg) in weight and 50 feet (15 m) tall by the age of 50 years! Obviously, there is a slowing of growth after the initial postnatal spurt although it is not entirely that

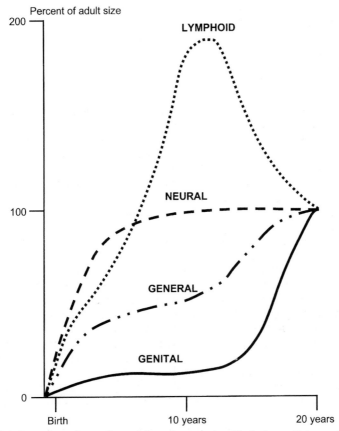

Figure 3.1 Comparison of rates of growth for main categories of body tissues. Note growth of the skull will be most influenced by the neural curve, whilst growth of the facial skeleton will more closely follow the general curve

simple: other growth spurts occur during childhood and different tissues grow at different rates and at different times. Figure 3.1, which is adapted from a diagram by Scammon (1930), shows the classic growth curves for the different tissues of the body. Obviously, the early acceleration in neural growth affects the growth of the skull (via the expansion of the brain) whilst the growth of the face mostly follows the general growth curve (somatic including skeletal). Having said this, there is some overlap of the two with, for example, the neural growth curve having a limited effect on the growth of the jaws, the maxilla being the most influenced. The overall effect of these differential patterns of tissue growth causes a change in body proportions over time, which is shown in Figure 3.2 and with which we are all familiar.

Figure 3.3 shows how one might expect the average individual to grow, with the early postnatal spurt followed by a smaller growth spurt about 6–8 years and a larger prepubertal spurt in the early teens. The latter is of particular relevance to the clinician employing treatment techniques that are largely growth dependent to treat a malocclusion (as an example of this see Chapter 18).

Although the majority of growth has been completed by 18 years of life there is good evidence that small increments of facial growth continue at least into the mid-thirties. This can affect both the shape and profile of the face whilst also having some influence in any later changes to the occlusion. However, the growth that one might expect after 16 years of age probably will have little

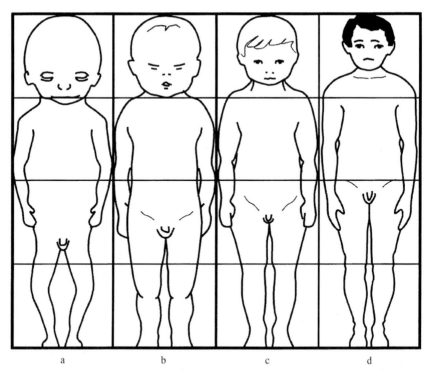

a   b   c   d

Figure 3.2 Change in body proportions with age. Note the gradual change in proportion of head from more than a quarter of body length in the four-month fetus (a); to just less than a quarter immediately post-birth (b); to approximately one-fifth of body length at two years of age (c). It is less than one-eighth of total length in the 14-year-old adolescent (d)

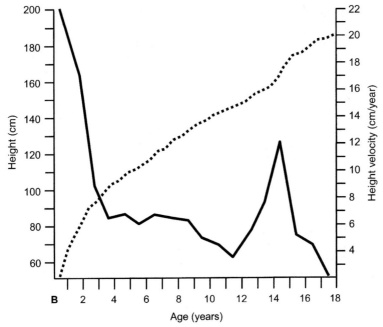

Figure 3.3 The normal growth process for the average individual: the gradual increase of height with time is plotted (dotted line) but more usefully the growth velocity is plotted against age (solid line). This shows the periods of maximum growth, termed growth 'spurts'

relevance when deciding on an orthodontic treatment plan. Therefore, a patient presenting after this age is probably best considered as an adult for the purposes of planning in this context (see Chapter 21).

Prenatal craniofacial growth and development

This may be divided into three stages:

1. The ovum – fertilization to 14th Day.
2. The embryo – 14th Day to 56th Day.
3. The fetus – 56th Day to birth.

Ovum: The first two weeks following fertilization consist of cell multiplication, cleavage and attachment to the uterine wall. The multiplying cells form a 'ball' just 1.5 mm across and there is little evidence of craniofacial differentiation at this stage.

Embryo: Between the second and third week *in utero* the embryo doubles in length and the differentiation of the head commences; at this stage the head is largely formed of prosencephalon and beneath the frontal process is the oral groove bounded laterally by the early maxillary processes. During the next four weeks a major part of the early facial development occurs, and the bucco-pharyngeal membrane, dividing the future oral cavity from the gut, ruptures. On either side of the frontal prominence ectoderm proliferates to form nasal placodes, which will become the future nasal epithelium. Between six and eight weeks, the maxillary processes grow forwards and mesially to unite with the lateral and medial nasal processes to initiate upper jaw development. Meanwhile beneath the maxillary processes are the developing pharyngeal pouches, which laterally form the branchial arches and grooves and are approximate to the lateral walls of the future pharynx.

Fetus: Between the second and third months *in utero* the length of the fetus increases three-fold, and all the facial structures become more pronounced with formation of nostrils and an increase in antero-posterior length of the maxilla and mandible. This is largely a period when change is related to an accelerated increase in size of the existing structures (growth) with changes in the relative proportions of those structures – for example relative enlargement of the jaws to the skull.

Growth of the face and skull

The cranium

Prenatal growth. The bones of the cranial vault develop in the membranes covering the brain in the embryo. The cranial vault forms initially by intra-membranous ossification within mesenchymal fibrocellular condensations and later in fetal life by proliferation and ossification of connective tissue at the sutures. The bones of the cranial vault are still well separated from each other at the end of the fetal stage by fontanelles, which facilitate movement of these bones to decrease skull size during passage down the birth canal.

Postnatal growth. Centres of ossification appear and the bones expand so that by birth they are related to one another at sutures, although in some areas – for example the fontanelles – there is still a membranous covering (Figure 3.4). The sutures are sites at which limited movement of the bones is possible and where growth in the size of the cranial vault can occur. They are fibrous joints with little inherent growth potential of their own. In fact growth at the sutures occurs by their expansion due to the increase in the volume of the cranial contents, which follows the neural growth pattern (see above). In addition to the increase in surface area, the bones of the cranial vault are thickened as a result of periosteal apposition. The cranial vault consists of outer and inner tables of compact bone separated by a layer of cancellous bone. Where functional demands require, for example at muscle attachments and sites of stress concentration, the outer table may be elevated into ridges and crests. This happens at the temporal and nuchal crests and at the supraorbital ridges where the space between the inner and outer tables becomes pneumatized.

The cranial base
The cranial base comprises the bones that develop from the cartilaginous chondrocranium of the embryo. By the end of the embryonic period the cranial base growth, originally related to an overall proliferation of cartilage, becomes (after the initiation of endochondral ossification), the responsibility of the proliferating, essentially cartilaginous, synchondroses. At birth, cartilage remains at these sites, where growth can occur to make adjustments in the future. The 'synchondroses' have a structure that resembles that of the epiphyseal

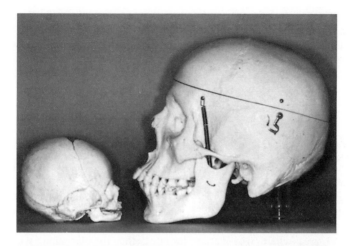

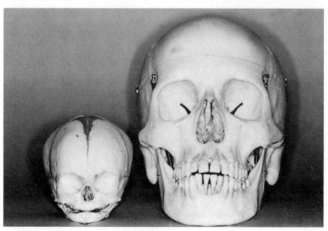

Figure 3.4 Neonate and adult skulls. Note the difference in proportions between the facial skeleton and the calvarium at the different ages. The proportions of the facial skeleton also change with age

cartilages of the long bones, except that, in this instance, growth occurs in both of the bones contributing to the joint. Two of these synchondroses persist later into childhood: the intersphenoidal (responsible for growth of the anterior skull base) closes at about seven years of age and the spheno-occipital (responsible for growth of the posterior skull base) closes in the late teens. Since there is little growth of the anterior cranial base after seven years this relatively stable area may be used as a reference structure on lateral skull radiographs from which growth changes elsewhere in the facial skeleton can be measured. When super-imposing radiographs this is better done as a 'best fit' around the ethmoid air sinuses rather than registering on either sella turcica or nasion (see Chapter 4). There are subtle remodelling changes that affect the shape of the sella during growth whilst there is forward movement of the outer table of bone at the nasion by a process of pneumatization.

The upper facial skeleton is related to the anterior cranial fossa whilst the mandible is related to the middle cranial fossa at its articulation with the temporal bone (Figure 3.5). Therefore, the length of the cranial base has an influence on jaw relationships, and growth at the spheno-occipital synchondrosis, which actively contributes until about the age of puberty, has a crucial influence on relative jaw position.

Growth of the cranial base cannot be influenced by orthodontic means and is probably under fairly tight genetic control.

The facial skeleton

The maxilla
Prenatal. The maxilla develops essentially as a membranous bone from two centres of ossification lateral to the nasal capsule in the maxillary processes of the first arch. Maxillary development is often described by dividing it into: the infraorbital area where ossification initiates; the alveolar area, where tooth development is important to local growth and development; and the frontal, zygomatic and palatal processes, which fan out from the centre of ossification. In addition there is development in cartilage, with subsequent ossification, in the paranasal processes of the nasal capsule and in areas at the alveolar border

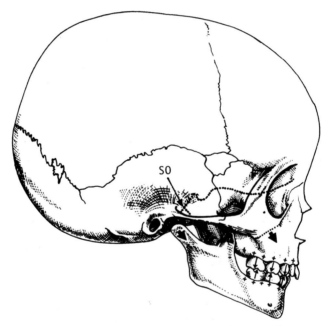

Figure 3.5 The maxilla grows downwards and forwards in part due to growth at sutures (i.e. displacement) and in part by surface apposition and remodelling of bone (i.e. drift). The mandible grows downwards and forwards from its cranial articulations at a greater rate than the maxilla. Thus the intermaxillary space grows in height and is bridged by vertical growth at the alveolar processes and eruption of the teeth. The midline cranial base is indicated by a dotted line. Growth at the spheno-occipital synchondrosis (SO) increases the distance between the cranial articulations of the maxilla and mandible

of the zygomatic process. It has been suggested that the primary cartilage of the nasal capsule is analogous to Meckel's cartilage, but it is certainly the precursor of the ethmoid and inferior turbinate bones.

There are some secondary cartilages present during early development of the maxilla, principally in the zygomatic process, but these have largely disappeared by the 12th week.

Following fusion of the maxilla and premaxilla at eight weeks *in utero* their growth is usually considered together.

Postnatal. The maxilla grows downwards and forwards from the anterior cranial base, partly as a result of growth at the circum-maxillary suture system, and partly as a result of extensive surface apposition and remodelling of bone. In general terms the outward and downward facing surfaces of the maxilla are formative, in particular at the alveolar process and on the oral surface of the palate, with corresponding resorption on the nasal surfaces. Thus the maxilla grows downwards and forwards partly due to drift (surface remodelling). The sutures of the upper facial skeleton are structurally comparable with those of the cranial vault and, like them, probably have little independent growth potential. However, it has not been possible to isolate the primary growth-promoting forces in the upper facial skeleton. Growth increments of the nasal septum and the eyeballs have been cited as possible factors but probably no single factor controls and directs growth of the upper facial skeleton. It has been shown that heavy forces applied to the maxillary teeth by orthodontic appliances can, according to the direction of traction, reduce or accelerate growth at the maxillary sutures. However, this is of limited practical application because, following such treatment, the natural growth pattern tends to reassert itself and there is a corresponding catch-up or lag so that the ultimate facial pattern is little affected. Only if such treatment were continued for many years, until facial growth was nearly complete, would lasting appreciable changes be achieved.

The mandible

Prenatal. As in other local structures, a considerable increase in growth of the mandible during the fetal period, especially in relation to length. Bone starts to form in a similar fashion to the maxilla about the primary cartilage and the local nerve – in this case Meckel's cartilage and the inferior dental nerve. Intramembranous ossification commences in fibrocellular condensations in these areas from about seven weeks *in utero*. The upper ends of Meckel's cartilage form the bones of the middle ear and are practically complete by 12 weeks. By birth most of Meckel's cartilage has gone except for small islands at the mental symphyses and spheno-mandibular and spheno-malleolar ligaments.

Ossification in the downward growing secondary (carrot) condylar cartilage (which developed at about the 12th week) appears to commence anteriorly in the fourth month of fetal life and by the end of the fifth month the only part of this cartilage left is beneath the articular surface of the condyle. This small residual area appears to be important in both later prenatal and postnatal growth and persists until the 20th year of life. Of the other secondary cartilages of the mandible that have been similarly present from the 12th week *in utero*, the coronoid cartilage disappears just before birth, having contributed to the process of the same name and the symphyseal cartilage disappears not long after, having contributed to the increase in width.

Postnatal. Growth in the overall length of the mandible takes place largely at the condyle but, of course, comparable remodelling periosteal growth changes take place to maintain the form of the mandible. It is an area of continuing controversy as to whether growth at the condyles propels the mandible downwards and forwards from the glenoid fossa or whether condylar growth is merely adaptive to other factors that carry the mandible downwards and forwards. Certainly, the growth of the mandible with its complex rotatory mechanisms would suggest a more sophisticated process to be at work. It seems probable that the condylar cartilage has an appreciable inherent growth potential but that it can be affected by local factors. However, its growth can be influenced only to a very limited extent by orthodontic appliance treatment. Proponents of functional appliances (see Chapter 18) claim that condylar growth can be controlled but this is still a matter of debate. The practitioner would be wise to plan treatment on the assumption that appliances will not influence condylar growth to any significant extent.

The mandible grows downwards and forwards from its articulation with the middle cranial fossa faster than does the maxilla (Figure 3.5). Antero-posteriorly this is largely compensated for by the growth of the spheno-occipital synchondrosis, which carries the maxilla forward. Again, bone surface deposition and resorption appear to play an important role in the translation and transposition of the mandible during postnatal growth. The precise nature of this process is perhaps best viewed diagrammatically in a more exhaustive text.

However, the tendency is for mandibular prognathism (i.e. projection from under the cranial structures) to increase slightly faster than maxillary prognathism.

Vertically the distance between the mandibular and maxillary bases – the intermaxillary space – increases. Vertical growth of the teeth and alveolar processes, which adapt to changes in height and shape of the intermaxillary space bridge this space.

The vertical relationship of the mandible to the upper facial structures is determined not only by growth at the condyles, but also by the lengths of the muscles and fasciae attached to it: principally the muscles of mastication, which pass between the mandible and the rest of the craniofacial skeleton, and the suprahyoid muscles below. Growth in length of these is, in turn, influenced by growth in length of the neck and the cervical vertebrae. Many other factors, such as the physiological need to maintain an airway, play a part in determining mandibular positions. This means that superimposed on the downward and forward translation of the mandible relative to the cranial base, there may be minor degrees of anterior or posterior rotation (Figure 3.6) depending on the balance of growth between the condyle and the muscles attached to the mandible. As discussed below, the positions of the teeth and alveolar structures adapt to these changes in mandibular relationships.

The palate

Prenatal. The primary palate is formed at about six weeks (*in utero*) from fusion of the mesially migrating maxillary processes with the lateral and medial nasal processes of the downward migrating fronto-nasal process. Failure of the fusion will lead to a cleft of the lip and primary palate. This may be either unilateral or bilateral (see Chapter 23).

The posterior palate derives from the vertically positioned palatal processes

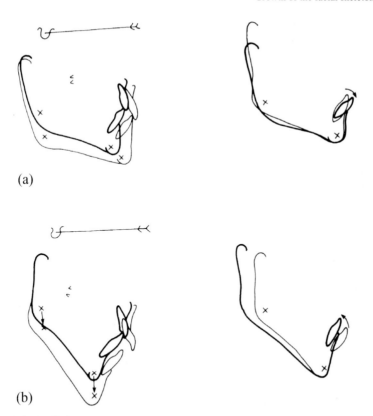

(a)

(b)

Figure 3.6 Mandibular growth rotations: (a) anterior (closing) growth rotation; (b) posterior (opening) growth rotation. The crosses indicate hypothetical stable points in the mandible, purely for the purposes of illustration. Where the posterior and anterior facial heights grow by different amounts a mandibular growth rotation will occur but will to a large extent be masked by remodelling at the lower and posterior borders of the mandible. This is revealed when mandibular outlines are superimposed on the stable structures. The relative orientation of the lower incisors within the face is usually maintained by dento-alveolar adaptation. In most children, growth rotations are small

or shelves of the developing maxilla. The tongue at this early stage of development is positioned between these shelves. However, at about 12 weeks (in the fetus stage) rapid forward and downward growth of the face occurs. This allows the tongue to take a more inferior position in the developing mouth, and the palatal shelves, by a largely unknown mechanism, move very rapidly, usually within 24 hours, up to a horizontal position. Subsequently, fusion in the midline, together with the nasal septum and primary palate, occurs to form the complete palate. Any disruption of this process may lead to failure of ectodermal fusion or failure of penetration of mesoderm across the centre line of the palate – either failure is likely to lead to a cleft palate.

Postnatal. After birth, growth in width of the palate occurs, partly at the mid-palatal suture (which can fuse in the early teens) and partly by differential bone resorption and desposition at the contralateral surfaces. The expansion of the mid-palatal suture also contributes to the width of the face in this area until its fusion.

Patterns of growth

At birth, the volume of the brain case is greater than that of the face (Figure 3.4), but after the age of six years there is little further growth in volume because the brain has nearly reached its adult size. The facial skeleton grows steadily over a much longer period and thus, in the adult, forms a much larger proportion of the skull than in the child, and projects further forwards from under the brain case (Figure 3.4). The infant face is relatively broad, but with postnatal growth the proportions of the face change, growth in breadth being least, and in depth most. Thus, on average, the face in an adult appears longer and narrower and projects further forwards than in the child (Figure 3.2).

Some of the more noticeable changes in facial characteristics are due to the fact that the eyes are relatively large in the infant but, like the brain, grow relatively little after the age of six years, whilst the nose is very much more prominent in the adult than in the child. These changes do not affect the occlusion, but changes in the character of the face obviously affect the appearance of the dentition in the face. Even with a 'normal' occlusion, the teeth of the nine-year-old child may seem to be rather large and prominent, but with growth of the rest of the face and in particular of the nose, the impression changes with time. Together with this trend it is apparent in Björk's growth studies, in which titanium implant markers had been placed in the basal bone of the jaws, that children's jaws become more prognathous with growth with a more pronounced chin button and anterior nasal spine. This anterior movement of the jaws forward is most pronounced in the mandible – hence the clinician's observation that: 'Class III malocclusions usually get worse with growth'.

It seems likely that this forward movement is related to the normal clockwise (closing) rotation of the jaws as they grow. If there is an 'over-rotation' a short lower facial height, prominent chin button and deep bite, Class II Division 2 malocclusion is often the result (Chapter 13). If the rotation is in the opposite direction (counterclockwise or opening) a long lower facial height and anterior open bite (long face) may be the result. The Burlington growth study observed the following average trends in facial growth:

- 85% are downwards and forwards
- 10% are vertical
- 5% are horizontal.

These trends may be interpreted in terms of the jaw growth rotations discussed earlier.

The control of facial growth

How is the force that displaces bones during growth both achieved and controlled? It would appear from what we have said so far that the periosteum and sutures and possibly also the condylar cartilage take a subordinate role during postnatal growth.

A possible hypothesis has been suggested by Moss. He suggests that bone is essentially a substance forming within capsules (surrounding sacks of soft tissue). These surrounding soft tissue 'sacs', by their growth and enlargement, determine the displacement of their encapsulated bones one from another. The position and growth of these soft tissues are, in turn, influenced by the functions that they perform and must maintain, an example being the airway. In other words, the soft tissues provide a growing 'functional matrix' within which the bones are displaced from one another; the space between these displaced (translated) bones is then 'filled in' by the laying down of bone by one means or another.

Certainly, this is an attractive philosophy – if one that is difficult to grasp immediately! It does at least provide a working hypothesis as to what may be the main displacing force in the growing face. However, this concept of growth does have problems. For example, it does not accommodate the observed behaviour of the cartilaginous primary growth centres like the long bone epiphysis, cranial base synchondrosis or nasal septal cartilage. These have all been shown to provide an independent 'force of growth' to displace the surrounding bone to accommodate newly ossified tissue.

However, when applied to the cranial vault, the functional matrix theory appears to work well. The bones of the skull exist in a capsule bound by the pia and dura mater. This matrix has the function of surrounding and covering the developing and growing brain. As the brain enlarges, the surrounding capsule enlarges and the bones within are displaced. The gaps created between the bones are then filled by the proliferating periosteum between them. The overall skull size thus increases. Certainly, skull growth closely matches the neural growth curve and this explains the very large skull, in comparison to the face, at birth and during the first couple of years of life – facial bone growth more closely follows the somatic curve of overall skeletal growth.

Therefore, it is easy to define areas of new bone formation and/or resorption during growth, whether by surface deposition beneath the periosteum, or at the suture, or by ossification of proliferating cartilage. It is less easy to be precise as to the nature of the force causing the displacement of the bones – the thrust of growth pushing the bones out into the environment. It may be concluded that no obvious overall control mechanism for facial growth has been identified thus far. It would appear that there is a complex of genetic and environmentally driven influences that determine the pattern and nature of growth but there is still much to be discovered in this area.

Growth spurts and kinetics

The different tissues of the body grow at different rates forming a variety of curves when the tissue size is plotted against time. Growth of the skeleton follows the general somatic growth pattern: there is an initial acceleration after birth, this then slows until there is another growth spurt between six and seven years of age. This acceleration may last for only 3–4 months and usually comes earlier in girls than boys. However, the spurt of most interest to orthodontists is the prepubertal acceleration. This again lasts just a few months, occurring (on average) at about 12 years in girls and 14 years in boys. There is a large variation in the timing (the standard deviation is one year), and it may occur as late as 16 years of age in some boys.

Average timing of growth spurts

Table 3.1 shows the average age during which an acceleration or spurt of growth may occur. Such spurts might last just 3–4 months. There is a 'three Ls' rule of growth in boys (in comparison to girls): usually they grow **L**ater – for **L**onger – and get **L**arger!

Table 3.1 **Average ages of growth spurts in boys and girls**

Mean age of 'spurt'	Girls	Boys
Early	Approx. 3 years	Approx. 3 years
Middle	6–7 years	7–9 years
Prepubertal	11–12 years	13–15 years

During the prepubertal period of rapid somatic growth there is some evidence that teeth move more rapidly in response to forces. In particular, certain appliance techniques are more effective: examples would be functional appliances (see Chapter 18) and extra-oral traction (see Chapter 17). For this reason attempts have been made to try and predict growth spurts in children so that treatment may be prescribed to coincide with these periods – such predictive techniques have so far proved to be unreliable.

It is also of some interest to clinicians to know when the majority of facial growth has ceased. This can affect the treatment planning (see Chapter 21) but is particularly important in the timing of orthognathic surgery (see Chapter 22). For the purposes of treatment planning, the majority of facial growth is usually complete by 16–17 years of age. Having said this, it is worth stating again that there is good evidence that small increments of facial growth occur into middle age. However, this is unlikely to be of any assistance (or relevance) in the treatment of malocclusion although it may contribute to any long-term process of relapse (see Chapter 25).

Facial growth and the occlusion

The alveolar bone is highly adaptable, depending for its existence and location on the presence and position of the teeth: remove a tooth and the associated alveolar process resorbs, move a tooth into the same area and it remodels.

Dento-alveolar compensation

Because the upper and lower teeth erupt into the 'neutral zone' of muscle balance between lips, cheeks and tongue they tend to be guided towards one another to establish an occlusion and to compensate for any transverse or antero-posterior malrelationships of the jaws. Variations in vertical jaw relationships are compensated, to a greater or lesser degree, on eruption of the teeth and growth of the alveolar processes. Where the skeletal malrelationships are too severe, the dento-alveolar compensation described above may not be sufficient to establish a normal occlusion and so crossbite, open bite and antero-posterior arch malrelationships may develop. However, arch malrelationships often will be less severe than might have been expected from the jaw malrelationship (see Figure 3.7).

In some cases dento-alveolar compensation does not operate because of variations in soft tissue patterns. For example, if the upper lip is short and the

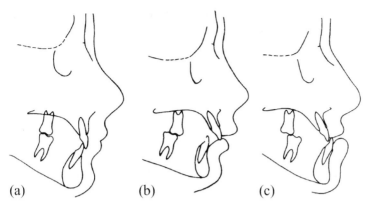

Figure 3.7 Skeletal patterns: (a) Class I; (b) Class II; (c) Class III

lips are habitually parted the upper incisors will tend to be proclined and are not guided towards the lower incisors. The lower incisors then will continue to erupt, possibly until they contact the palate.

Dento-alveolar compensation is not always advantageous: in some cases of mandibular retrusion, for example, compensation occurs by retroclination of the upper incisors (see Figure 12.3). This type of incisor relationship is usually associated with a deep overbite and may, when associated with poor oral hygiene, be traumatic as well as being unsightly.

Dento-alveolar adaptation

As the face grows, the intermaxillary space increases in height and the antero-posterior jaw relationship may change. As a result of vertical growth of the teeth and alveolar processes, occlusal contacts, and the soft tissue environment of the teeth, the existing occlusion or malocclusion tends to be maintained. Dento-alveolar adaptation is a dynamic process whilst dento-alveolar compensation refers to an existing state of affairs: on examining a patient, it is possible to ascertain to what extent dento-alveolar compensation exists. Only with records obtained on more than one occasion can one identify the nature and amount of dento-alveolar adaptation that may have occurred over that time period.

Dento-alveolar adaptation is greatest vertically, in response to vertical growth of the intermaxillary space. Little change in transverse jaw relationships occurs with growth. Where changes in antero-posterior jaw relationships occur there will usually be a corresponding dento-alveolar adaptation. Most commonly the mandible grows forwards slightly more than the maxilla and the upper incisors procline whilst the lower incisors retrocline. The proclination of the upper incisors does not produce spacing because the upper buccal segments come forwards by a comparable amount. Retroclination of the lower incisors usually results in crowding. If the adaptive mechanisms cannot cope with the extent of the change in jaw relationships there will be occlusal change. This most often happens where there is a Class III arch relationship (see Figure 3.7c) and there is little or no incisor overbite.

Growth rotations of the mandible may be superimposed upon the changes described above. Such growth rotations initiate dento-alveolar adaptation, which may in turn lead to lower incisor crowding. With a posterior (opening) growth rotation (Figure 3.6b) the lower incisors tend to become retroclined under the influence of the soft tissue integument of the face so that their relationship to upper facial reference planes changes very little. The buccal segments do not move back by a corresponding amount and so lower arch crowding may appear or become more severe.

Anterior mandibular (closing) growth rotations (Figure 3.6a) are associated with proclination of the lower incisors within the alveolar process and with an upward and forward path of eruption of the buccal teeth. Measured to a reference plane in the upper face, the lower incisors do not become proclined but maintain their inclination. Provided that the forward movement of anterior and posterior teeth are in balance there should be no change in the space conditions of the lower arch. However, the lower incisors, through contact with the upper incisors, are often prevented from adapting completely, particularly if at the same time the mandible is growing forwards to a greater extent than the maxilla. In these circumstances the lower buccal teeth will encroach on space for the lower labial segment with the development of lower incisor crowding.

Growth changes during treatment

Orthodontic treatment planning for the child is based on the hypothesis that the growth changes which take place will be within the normal range and so will have only minor effects on the shape of the facial skeleton and thus the occlusion. This is satisfactory for the majority of patients but occasionally unforeseen changes may occur and treatment planning may have to be revised. Many attempts have been made to predict accurately the future growth trends of the facial skeleton in the individual, but at the present time this is not possible.

Prediction of the pattern of facial growth

Occasionally facial profiles and malocclusions may worsen or improve with facial growth; obviously in such individuals it would be an advantage to predict such changes in the facial pattern.

Methods have been suggested whereby growth increments occur at different parts of the jaws to simulate average yearly growth – in its crudest form this has involved the use of a clear acetate template, while more sophisticated approaches involve the use of a computer database. Whichever approach is used, although reasonable at predicting the average 'grower', such simulation methods are currently not reliable in predicting the 'abnormal grower' – the patient in whom the orthodontist might be most interested.

Another approach has been from the genetic viewpoint using a comparison of family likeness in siblings and other relations together with a suitable formula to predict the facial type. This might, for instance, work well in predicting the lower jaw size of a member of the Hapsburg royal family, who were famous for their characteristically large lower jaw. However, usually by nine years of age the face is 85% of its adult size and thus such a growth trend would be better predicted by the current appearance of the patient without any further assessment.

Other methods for growth prediction have been suggested but the present 'state of the art' is that only average growth trends may be predicted within an acceptable margin of error.

The uncertainty of facial growth prediction is magnified in those patients with a craniofacial disruption, of which cleft lip and palate is an obvious example.

Normal growth

It is difficult to be precise as to what constitutes normal growth. For example, if one is using height as the appropriate yardstick, and a sample of 12-year-old children are examined, one will find a large range or variation about the norm or mean. Factors determining growth may be broadly divided into genetic and environmental – the relative importance of each in any individual is often difficult to determine.

It has been suggested that 'growth is the meeting point of heredity and environment' but where that meeting point is precisely located is less easy to define. Certainly, hereditary factors are important in determining the facial form when considering family or racial likeness. However, hereditary factors are tempered by the environment, the socioeconomic background, and the quality of the diet, the health of a community, or individual soft tissue adaptations or habits.

In the final analysis it is not important for the clinician to be able to define what is normal but rather to be able to identify what may constitute the abnormal.

Further reading

Behrents, R.G. (1985). *Growth in the Ageing Craniofacial Skeleton*. Ann Arbor: University of Michigan. Center for Human Growth & Development.

Björk, A. (1968). The use of metallic implants in the study of facial growth in children: method and application. *American Journal of Physical Anthropology*, **29**, 243–50.

Enlow, D.H. (1990). *Handbook of Facial Growth*, 3rd edn. Philadelphia: W.B. Saunders.

Houston, W.J.B. (1979). The current status of facial growth prediction: a review. *British Journal of Orthodontics*, **6**, 11–17.

Houston, W.J.B. (1980). Relationships between skeletal maturity estimated from hand–wrist radiographs and the timing of the adolescent growth spurt. *European Journal of Orthodontics*, **2**, 81–93.

Koski, K. (1968). Cranial growth centres: facts or fallacies? *American Journal of Orthodontics*, **54**, 566–83.

Moss, M.L. (1969). The primary role of functional matrices in facial growth. *American Journal of Orthodontics*, **55**, 566–77.

Mossey, P.A. (1999). The heritability of malocclusion: parts I & II. *British Journal of Orthodontics*, **2**, 103–13; 156–66.

Proffit, W.R. (ed.) (2000). Concepts of growth and development. In *Contemporary Orthodontics*, 2nd edn, pp. 24–62. St Louis: Mosby Yearbook.

Scammon, R.E. (1930). The measurement of the body in childhood. In *The Measurement of Man* (J.A. Harris, ed.) Minneapolis, MN: University of Minnesota Press.

Sperber, G.H. (1996). Craniofacial embryology. In *Dental Practitioner Handbook*, 4th edn. London: Wright.

Chapter 4

Analysis of the facial skeleton

The skeletal relationship: clinical considerations

The relationship between the jaws has important effects on dental arch relationship. Unless lateral skull radiographs are available (see Figure 4.2), jaw relationship is assessed from the clinical examination of the patient. Skeletal relationships should be considered in three axes: antero-posterior, vertical and transverse.

Clinical assessment

Antero-posterior
This sagittal relationship between the jaws (the skeletal pattern) depends on the length of the maxilla, length of mandible and the length of the cranial base between its articulation with the maxilla and the temporomandibular joint. The skeletal pattern is assessed by examining the profile as the patient sits unsupported, with the head in the free postural position and the mandible in the rest position or with the teeth in centric occlusion (the mandible must not be postured or displaced). When the mandible is normally related to the maxilla the skeletal pattern is Class I; when it is posteriorly positioned relative to the maxilla the skeletal pattern is Class II; and when it is too far forward the skeletal pattern is Class III (see Figure 3.7). Subjective assessment of this sort is open to error and if there is a marked discrepancy between the thickness of the upper and lower lips, or a prominent chin 'button' (pogonion) the soft tissue profile

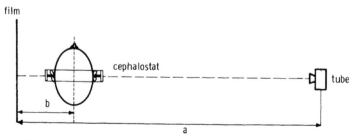

Figure 4.1 When a cephalometric radiograph is obtained, the head is held in a fixed relationship to the film and X-ray source (tube). The ratio a/b determines the enlargement of the image

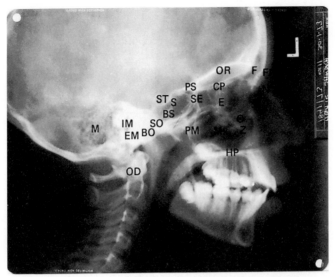

Figure 4.2 A lateral skull radiograph illustrating the principal anatomical features. Note: for purposes of reproducibility and accuracy these are most usefully taken with the head held in a cephalostat (as in Figure 4.1)

BO = basi-occiput
BS = basi-sphenoid
CP = cribriform plate of ethmoid
E = ethmoid air cells
EM = external acoustic meatus
F = frontal sinus
FN = fronto-nasal suture
HP = hard palate
IM = internal acoustic meatus
M = mastoid air cells
Mx = maxillary sinus
N = nasal bones

O = orbital margins
OD = odontoid process of axis
OR = orbital roof
PM = pterygomaxillary fissure
PS = planum sphenoidale
S = sphenoid air sinus
SE = spheno-ethmoidal synchondrosis
SO = spheno-occipital synchondrosis
ST = sella turcica, the pituitary fossa
Z = zygomatic process of maxilla

may give a misleading impression of the skeletal pattern. Nevertheless, this method of assessment is usually more accurate than attempts to judge skeletal relationships with the lips retracted. Minor variations in skeletal pattern are of little clinical importance and the larger variations from normal, which do have a bearing on aetiology and treatment, can readily be recognized.

Vertical
The space between the upper and lower skeletal bases is the intermaxillary space. The height of this space depends on the shape of the mandible and on the resting lengths of the muscles of mastication. Where the anterior height of the intermaxillary space is large an open bite may be found (Chapter 8).

The angle between the Frankfort and mandibular planes (Figure 4.3) gives an index of anterior intermaxillary height. The average value for this angle is 27°, with a normal range of 5° in either direction. If the Frankfort–mandibular planes angle is large the anterior intermaxillary height will usually be increased. It is not easy to estimate by eye the size of the Frankfort–mandibular planes angle.

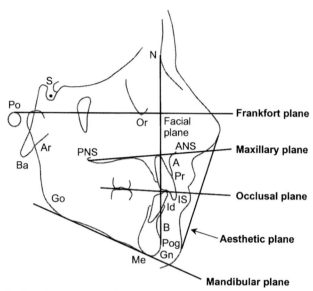

Figure 4.3 Tracing of the radiograph shown in Figure 4.2, indicating the main cephalometric landmarks (see text for definitions of abbreviations)

Various forms of protractor are available but it is perhaps simpler to compare the lower facial height – menton to anterior nasal spine (ANS) – to the middle facial height – ANS to nasion (Figure 4.3). In the well-balanced face these heights should be approximately equal. Clearly, the ratio between them will be affected by mid-facial height but a relative increase in lower facial height may be associated with a skeletal open bite.

Transverse
The relative widths of the jaws have a bearing on the transverse relationship of the dental arches (Chapter 10). However, there is no way, clinically or radio-logically, in which these widths can be accurately measured. Discrepancies in skeletal base width usually have to be inferred from transverse malrelationships of the arches.

Facial asymmetry
Whilst no face is perfectly symmetrical, significant differences from the norm should be apparent by careful clinical examination. Asymmetries usually occur due to discrepancies in growth between the left and right sides in one or more of the facial dimensions mentioned above. Generally, abnormal asymmetries of the face may be assessed by comparison of one side of the face to the other, any resultant cant in the occlusion can be more clearly observed by getting the patient to occlude, in the region of the molars, across a wooden tongue spatula.

A good way to assess facial asymmetry is to rest the chair back and view the patient from above, looking at the relationship of forehead, nose and chin-point. Always look for displacements on mandibular closure in these patients, which can exaggerate the asymmetry of the chin.

Cephalometric analysis

Analysis of lateral skull radiographs allows a more detailed evaluation of facial structures than is possible from a visual assessment of facial appearance. The cephalometric lateral skull radiograph (lateral cephalogram) is taken with the head held in a specially designed holder (Figure 4.1) so that there is a fixed constant relationship between the patient's head, the film and the anode of the X-ray tube. The mid-sagittal plane of the head should be parallel to and at a fixed distance from the film so that linear measurements are magnified by a known standard amount (usually about 10%). To get consistent posing of the patient's head the patient may be asked to look at an 'imagined' horizon or look into a mirror, or a small spirit level may be employed. Some experience is required if a lateral cephalogram radiograph is to be interpreted reliably. The features shown in Figures 4.2 and 4.3 give a key to the general anatomy. Cephalometric landmarks can then be located (Figure 4.3). The appearance of each landmark can vary appreciably between patients, and some are much more difficult to identify reliably than others. If the film is overexposed it can be very difficult to locate the fine bony detail on the skeletal profile.

Definitions of landmarks (Figure 4.3)

Note: definitions using 'lowest' or 'highest' assume that the radiograph is orientated so that the Frankfort plane is horizontal.

Anterior nasal spine (ANS). The point of the bony nasal spine. The vertical level can be fixed quite reliably but the antero-posterior location may be difficult: the tip of the spine is thin and nasal cartilages, which are nearly of the same radio-opacity, may overlay it. Harvold recommended the use of points on the lower and upper contours of the spine where it was 3 mm thick. These may be more reliable than the traditional ANS but they may still be difficult to locate because the upper and lower margins of the spine are not always distinct.

Articulare (Ar). The point of intersection of the projection of the surface of the neck of the condyle and the inferior surface of the basi-occiput.

Basion (Ba). The most posterior inferior point in the midline on the basi-occiput. This marks the posterior limit of the midline cranial base and lies on the anterior rim of the foramen magnum.

Gonion (Go). The most posterior, inferior point on the angle of the mandible. It is located by drawing tangents to the angle of the mandible through the menton and through the articulare. The gonion lies where the bisector of the angle formed by these two tangents intersects the mandibular outline. This point may be used in drawing the mandibular plane and gonial angle. Where the outlines of the two sides do not coincide an 'average' outline should be drawn and the constructions related to this.

Gnathion (Gn). The most anterior, inferior point on the bony symphysis of the mandible. It is located where the bisector of the angle between the facial line (NPog) and the mandibular plane (through menton and tangent to the angle of the mandible) intersects the outline of the symphysis.

Incision inferius (II). The tip of the crown of the most prominent mandibular incisor.

Incision superius (IS). The tip of the crown of the most prominent maxillary incisor.

Infradentale (Id). The highest point on the alveolar crest labial to the most prominent lower incisor.

Menton (Me). The lowermost point on the mandibular symphysis.

Nasion (N). The most anterior point on the fronto-nasal suture.

Orbitale (Or). The most inferior point on the margin of the orbit. Strictly speaking, the left orbit should be used and some orthodontists use a radio-opaque pointer, or fix a marker to the skin before the radiograph is taken, to indicate this. When this is not done and two orbital borders are shown, the midpoint should be taken. The orbitale is difficult to locate with accuracy.

Posterior nasal spine (PNS). The tip of the posterior nasal spine can usually be seen unless unerupted molars obscure it. The outline of the palate gives a good indication of its vertical level and allows the maxillary plane to be drawn in. A line through the most inferior point on the pterygomaxillary fissure, perpendicular to the maxillary plane, indicates the antero-posterior location of PNS.

Pogonion (Pog). The most anterior point of the bony chin.

Point A (A). Also known as subspinale, this is the deepest point on the maxillary profile between the anterior nasal spine and the alveolar crest. It can be difficult to locate if the maxillary profile is not clear: there may be a thin spine of bone extending downwards in the midline from the anterior nasal spine, or the shadow of the cheek can be superimposed. Point A is used to indicate the anterior limit of the maxillary base but it is not very reliable in this respect because the bone in this region remodels to some extent with orthodontic tooth movement, quite apart from the problems of locating the point. However, in spite of these difficulties, point A continues to be used because no entirely satisfactory alternative has been proposed.

Point B (B). Also known as supramentale, this is the mandibular point that corresponds to point A on the maxilla; however, it is more reliable. It is the deepest point on the concavity of the mandibular profile between the point of the chin and the alveolar crest. If the curvature is gentle, the vertical level of point B may be difficult to fix, but this is not usually very important because it is used to measure antero-posterior jaw relationships.

Porion (Po). The highest point on the bony external acoustic meatus. If both sides are visible, the midpoint is taken. As already mentioned, the porion can be very difficult to locate reliably. A useful guide is that the upper borders of the external acoustic meatus should be on the same level as the articulating surfaces of the mandibular condyles, although these too are difficult to locate. Others have suggested using the highest point on the earpost of the cephalostat, although this may vary with soft tissue compression of the ear.

Prosthion (Pr). The lowest point on the alveolar crest labial to the most prominent upper central incisor.

Sella (S). The mid-point of the sella turcica.

Reference lines and planes (Figures 4.3 and 4.4)

Cephalometric measurements will be described with the analyses, but certain widely used reference planes (or more correctly 'lines' as we are dealing with a two-dimensional representation) will be described here. A very large number of reference lines in the skull are described in the anthropological literature, but only a few of direct orthodontic importance will be mentioned.

Facial line (or plane). Nasion–pogonion. It indicates the general orientation of the facial profile.

Frankfort plane. Porion–orbitale. This plane is described as being horizontal when the head is in a free postural position. In fact, there is considerable individual variation. This, together with the unreliability of its end points and the fact that it represents no single coherent anatomical structure, means that there are serious reservations about its use as a reference structure.

Mandibular plane (Mn). A variety of lines have been used to indicate the orientation of the body of the mandible, but which one is selected probably makes little difference. The simplest to locate is the line from the menton, tangent to the lower border of the mandible at the angle. The line Go–Gn is used by many but requires the construction of both points.

Maxillary plane (Mx). This line through the anterior and posterior nasal spines indicates the orientation of the palate. Where the anterior nasal spine curves upwards above the level of the nasal floor, it may be better to draw the maxillary plane through the PNS parallel to the nasal floor.

Occlusal plane. Various definitions are offered. It may be represented by the line that passes through the occlusion of the mesial cusps of the most anterior permanent molars and halfway between the tips of the upper and lower central incisors. It is preferable to use a line following the occlusion of the molar and premolar teeth. This is known as the functional occlusal plane (FOP).

Many landmarks are a compromise between anatomical validity and the possibility of identification. For example, points A and B, which are meant to represent the maxillary and mandibular skeletal base respectively, are affected to a limited extent by tooth movement and alveolar remodelling. Thus cephalometric measurements must be interpreted with caution and too much emphasis should not be placed on minor variations in their values. If a cephalometric measurement is to have any meaning it is necessary to know the normal range of that measurement within the population group from which the patient comes (see Figure 4.4). Even if one measurement is beyond the normal range it may be compensated for by other features and so it is necessary to look for a general pattern. The basic question is whether there is evidence of skeletal malrelationships and whether or not there has been dento-alveolar compensation. It is then possible to decide about the tooth movements that would be necessary to correct the arch malrelationships; and whether tipping movements (obtainable with a

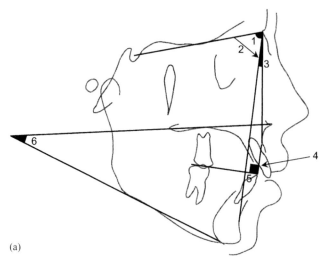

(a)

Figure 4.4 (a) and (b) A typical cephalometric analysis

	Mean	Range + or −	This case
1. SNA	82 degrees	3	79 degrees
2. SNB	79 degrees	3	72 degrees
3. ANB	3 degrees	1	7 degrees
4. AB/FOP	90 degrees	5	100 degrees
5. A/B perp. FOP (Wit's)	0 mm	3	8 mm
6. Max./Mand. Planes (MM)	27 degrees	5	29 degrees
7. U1/Max. Plane	108 degrees	5	110 degrees
8. L1/Mand. Plane	92 degrees	5	102 degrees
9. U1/L1	133 degrees	10	119 degrees
10. L1 to A–Pog	0 mm	2	+4 mm
11. Upper lip to Aesthetic plane	0 mm	−	+1 mm
12. Lower lip to Aesthetic plane	0 mm	−	+4 mm

Comments: Angle SNA is low but just within normal range whilst SNB is definitely low. Angle ANB at 7 degrees indicates a definite Class II skeletal pattern and this is corroborated by the large angle between the line A–B and the functional occlusal plane (FOP). Another method of examining the skeletal pattern is Wit's analysis: measuring the difference at the FOP of perpendiculars from A and B points. In this case a significant Class II discrepancy is shown. A normal reading would be 0 mm for females and B perp. + 1 mm for males. The upper incisors are at an average inclination to the maxillary plane whilst the lower incisors are proclined with the incisor edges in advance of the A–Pog line, indicating some dento-alveolar compensation for the Class II skeletal pattern. Vertically the jaw relationships are within normal limits. The lips were parted when the radiograph was taken, with the lower lip rather full and everted lying in advance of the Aesthetic Plane. It is important to assess clinically whether this correctly portrays the habitual lip posture

removable appliance) or controlled apical movement (requiring fixed appliances) will be appropriate. Where the skeletal discrepancy is severe, surgical correction may be considered.

Treatment planning must never be undertaken using cephalometric analysis in isolation: the stability and aesthetic acceptability of the intended tooth movements can be fully evaluated only by reference to the soft tissue pattern and facial appearance of the 'live patient'.

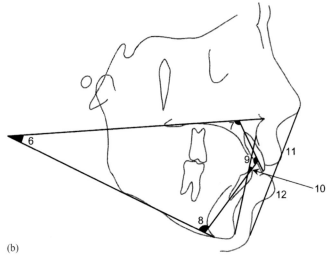

(b)

Figure 4.4 *Continued*

Measurement from lateral skull radiographs

The relevant anatomical lines should be traced on to good quality tracing paper using a sharp, hard pencil. A very large number of cephalometric measurements have been proposed but, for the clinician, those shown in Figure 4.4 give a comprehensive view of skeletal and dento-skeletal relationships.

Electronic digitizers linked to a computer applying a suitable software package are used increasingly for cephalometric analysis. Such a system speeds the whole process whilst facilitating the application of more than one method of analysis. This is particularly useful in cases requiring orthognathic surgery. The software allows manipulation of the image on the monitor to assess the effects of different surgical procedures. Newly developed systems allow the merger of video-captured images of the patient together with the appropriate radiograph, but these are still expensive. Although not always accurate, such systems can help both clinicians and patients visualize the likely effects of various treatment options.

The interpretation of cephalometric measurements

Points A and B are taken to represent the anterior limits of the tooth-bearing areas of the maxilla and mandible. This relationship is usually assessed by reference to the anterior cranial base (S–N line). Angles SNA and SNB measure the prognathism, or projection, in relation to the cranial base, of the maxilla and mandible. The difference between these (angle ANB) gives an indication of the jaw relationships (Table 4.1).

Table 4.1   Relationship between ANB angle and skeletal classification

ANB Angle	Skeletal classification
2–4 degrees	I
>4 degrees	II
<2 degrees	III

This ANB value can be misleading if the position of N is unusual but a warning of this may be given by a value of SNA that is unusually large or small. An alternative method of assessing the jaw relationship is to measure the angle between A and B and the functional occlusal plane (FOP). Perpendicular lines may also be dropped from these points to the occlusal plane (Wit's analysis). A problem with both measurements is that the orientation of the FOP varies greatly between individuals and can change with growth and treatment. However, they offer a useful check on the information given by angle ANB: if different evaluations of the skeletal pattern are contradictory, then each should be interpreted with caution and a final judgement on skeletal relationships made from clinical observations.

As with direct clinical observation the anterior height of the intermaxillary space may be estimated from the angle of the mandibular plane to the Frankfort plane, but as the latter is often difficult to locate on a radiograph the maxillary plane (ANS–PNS) is often used instead. On average, the Frankfort and maxillary planes are parallel to one another but they may diverge appreciably in some individuals.

Dento-skeletal relationships

The inclinations of the upper incisors to the maxillary plane and of the lower incisors to the mandibular plane give an indication of whether or not any dento-alveolar compensation for antero-posterior skeletal discrepancies has taken place (see Figure 22.5). They also give a guide to the type of tooth movements that will be required to correct incisor malrelationships. The distance of the most prominent lower incisor from the line between point A and the chin point (pogonion) is a guide to the position of the lower incisors relative to the lower skeletal profile. It is simpler to obtain a good incisor relationship, and the appearance is usually better if the lower incisor edge lies close to the A–Po line than if it is far from it. However, this line should not be regarded as a treatment goal to the positioning of the lower incisors because it offers no guide to the position of stability.

The angle between the upper and lower incisors is related to the depth of overbite (except in Class III cases). A wide interincisor angle is usually associated with a deep overbite and if at the end of treatment this angle remains large, the overbite will usually deepen and may become traumatic.

The soft tissue profile

Various cephalometric assessments of the soft tissue profile have been proposed. It must be recognized that none of these can give guidance as to whether a particular face is attractive or not and such measurements are of very little diagnostic value. However, they may help in describing a patient's facial appearance. Perhaps the most useful of these is the Aesthetic Line, which touches the tip of the nose and the tip of the chin. It has been maintained that the facial appearance is more likely to be pleasing when the lips lie close to this line. Another indicator is the naso-labial angle: ideally the naso-labial angle should be of the order of 110°. Too obtuse (large) a naso-labial angle often gives a rather poor facial appearance. Careful consideration should be given to the management of patients with a tendency towards a more obtuse naso-labial angle: reduction of an overjet, particularly with a fixed appliance, can have undesirable effects on the lip profile.

Racial variation

Note that the norm values given in Figure 4.4 have been derived from Caucasian groups and should not be applied to other racial groups.

Postero-anterior or frontal cephalograms

It is also possible to take jaw and skull radiographs using a cephalostat to produce a postero-anterior view. However, such films are difficult to reproduce consistently and point identification is generally inaccurate. On occasions they may aid the assessment of a clinically diagnosed facial asymmetry but are of limited use in any detailed analysis.

In patients with severe craniofacial asymmetry, often syndromal in origin, three dimensional radiographic **CAT** scans may be taken (see Chapter 19). However, significant radiation dosages to the patient are associated with the taking of such computer-based images. As a consequence they should only be considered prior to a likely joint orthodontic/surgical treatment. Such data can be used to generate CAD/CAM acrylic models of a patient's skull and jaws for detailed surgical planning.

Less invasive light scanning systems are under current evaluation. They can capture three dimensional images of the face and will be of great value in the future in the diagnosis and treatment of facial deformity.

Further reading

Baumrind, S. and Frantz, R.C. (1971). The reliability of head film measurements. 1) Landmark identification. *American Journal of Orthodontics*, **60**, 111–27.

Baumrind, S. and Frantz, R.C. (1971). The reliability of head film measurements. 2) Conventional angular and linear measurements. *American Journal of Orthodontics*, **60**, 505–17.

Broadbent, B.H. (1931). A new X-ray technique and its application to orthodontics. *Angle Orthodontist*, **1**, 45–66.

Broadbent, B.H. (1937). The face of the normal child: Bolton standards and technique. *Angle Orthodontist*, **7**, 183–233.

Downs, W. B. (1948). Variations in facial relationships; their significance in treatment and prognosis. *American Journal of Orthodontics*, **34**, 812–40.

Gravely, J.F. and Benzies, P.M. (1974). The clinical significance of tracing error in cephalometry. *British Journal of Orthodontics*, **1**, 95–101.

Houston, W.J.B. (1983). The analysis of errors in orthodontic measurements. *American Journal of Orthodontics*, **83**, 382–90.

Jacobson, A. (1975). The 'Wits' appraisal of jaw disharmony. *American Journal of Orthodontics*, **67**, 125–33.

Chapter 5

The soft tissues: morphology and behaviour

Traditionally the soft tissues considered to have greatest influence on tooth positions have been the lips and the tongue, with the emphasis being placed on their respective functions during swallowing. However, the current view that teeth will move optimally in response to light continuous forces suggests that the resting positions of tongue and lips are of greater significance in dictating tooth position than the transient heavy forces exerted during swallowing. It is important to remember that other soft tissues of the mouth and naso-pharynx, such as the fraenum, periodontal ligament and adenoidal tissues, may also have a role in the aetiology of malocclusion and the stability of orthodontic treatment.

Muscle balance

The teeth occupy a position of balance determined by the interaction between the tongue and lips, the jaw relationship and occlusal forces. If the position of the teeth is to be altered and remain stable, another position of balance must be sought. Alteration of the balance of soft tissue forces, by relieving the pressures of the cheeks and lips while allowing the tongue to expand the dental arches laterally and antero-posteriorly, is deliberately attempted by the exponents of some myofunctional appliances (see Chapter 18).

The lips

The lips may be described as being either competent or incompetent.

Competent lips

In this situation the lips are held together easily, with minimal activity of the circumoral musculature, forming an anterior oral seal when the mandible is in the rest position (Figure 5.1a).

In patients where the lips have the potential to meet easily together, but are held apart, the term potentially competent may be applied. This may be found in those patients where prominent upper incisors rest between the lips or where nasal obstruction encourages mouth breathing.

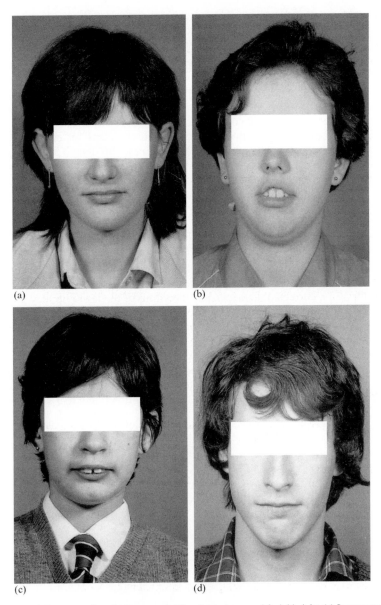

Figure 5.1 (a) Competent lips. (b) Incompetent lips due to increased facial height. (c) Incompetent lips due to severe antero-posterior skeletal discrepancy. (d) Incompetent lips held together by muscular effort; note the puckering of the skin over the chin signifying mentalis muscle activity

Incompetent lips

In this situation, where there is minimal activity of the circumoral musculature and the mandible in the rest position, the lips are held apart. In the absence of any neuromuscular deficit, such as that found in cerebral palsy, this is usually due to an imbalance between the anterior lower face height and the length of the upper and lower lips (Figure 5.1b) or a severe antero-posterior discrepancy (Figure 5.1c).

The degree of incompetence varies between individuals, depending on both their skeletal and dental architecture. Mild or moderately incompetent lips may be held together with muscular effort. This can be recognized by the puckering of the skin over the chin due to the contraction of the mentalis muscle (Figure 5.1d). In more severe cases the patient will have great difficulty in achieving even transitory lip contact.

Lip exercises (which are prescribed by some clinicians for use with certain types of functional appliances) will not increase lip length, but they may encourage the development of a neuromuscular habit that brings the lips together. Such changes may be difficult to distinguish from those that are often seen to occur naturally as the child matures.

Significance of lips

It has been suggested that the lower lip has an important role in the development of a malocclusion, in treatment to correct a malocclusion and in the long-term stability of the corrected malocclusion. The form of the lower lip may guide the path of the erupting permanent incisors. In patients with a reduced anterior lower face height, the lower lip may direct the erupting maxillary incisors down its inner surface and contribute to the establishment of a Class II Division 2 malocclusion, or alternatively it may guide the incisors labially to produce a Class II Division 1 malocclusion. Of course, the developmental position of the incisors is also an important contributory factor and the interrelationship between soft and hard tissues is complex. Clinically it is found that where the lips

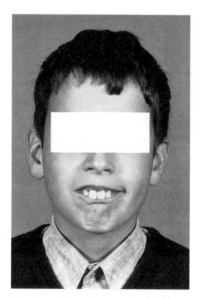

Figure 5.2 Tongue to lower lip oral seal. Note the upper lip plays no part in forming an anterior oral seal. The activity of the lower lip will hinder the overjet reduction

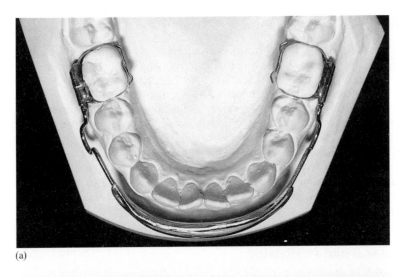

(a)

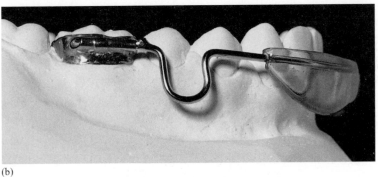

(b)

Figure 5.3 A lip bumper being used to harness muscular forces from the lower lip in order to move lower molars distally. (a) Occlusal view; (b) right buccal view

are full and everted both the upper and lower labial segments are more often proclined (bimaxillary proclination), whereas in individuals with more vertically positioned or straight lips the upper and lower labial segments are more often retroclined (bimaxillary retroclination).

During treatment of a Class II Division 1 malocclusion, the contact of lower lip to tongue to form an oral seal may make overjet reduction difficult (Figures 5.2 and 12.2a). On occasions muscular activity of the lower lip may be harnessed by means of a lip bumper to help move lower teeth distally (Figure 5.3a,b).

The long-term stability of a corrected Class II Division 1 malocclusion relies on the lower lip covering the incisal third of the labial surface of the upper incisors to control their position (see Figure 12.2b). If this treatment aim cannot be achieved there is a risk that without permanent or semipermanent retention of upper incisor position the overjet will re-establish.

The tongue

The tongue adapts to the form of the oral cavity. In the infant the tongue lies between the gum pads in contact with the lips and cheeks. Feeding and swallowing take place with the tongue in this forward position. As the teeth erupt oral function changes, mastication is established and there is a gradual maturation of tongue activity from infantile to a more adult pattern. This is usually complete by the time the deciduous dentition has become established. However, for a small number of individuals the infantile pattern of behaviour may persist and influence the position of incisor teeth.

Lateral spread of the tongue, especially in the lower arch, has been suggested as the mechanism that prevents the first permanent molar from moving mesially as much when both deciduous molars have been extracted, as when a single deciduous second molar has been lost (Figure 5.4).

Oral seal and swallowing

The tongue will usually work in conjunction with the lower lip to form an anterior oral seal, both at rest and during swallowing.

Oral seal

This may be found in different circumstances, as outlined below:

- Where the lips are incompetent and habitually parted, an anterior oral seal

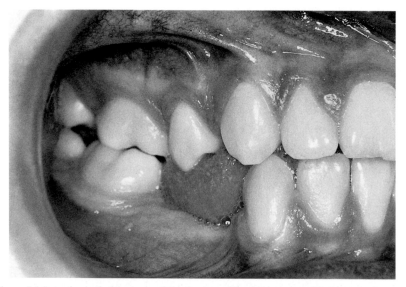

Figure 5.4 Lateral spread of the tongue following loss of the first and second deciduous molars preventing substantial mesial movement of the lower first permanent molar. Note also that there has been no over-eruption of the opposing premolar

may be obtained by contact between the tongue and lower lip. This will be associated with an incomplete overbite and some upper incisor proclination.

- A large overjet such as is found in a Class II skeletal pattern will lead to an anterior oral seal by tongue/lower lip contact. The features are similar to those associated with incompetent lips (above).
- If the overbite is incomplete, due for example to a digit-sucking habit or an increased lower face height, the tongue will come forwards over the lower incisors. As with all adaptive characteristics this will spontaneously revert to normal on correction of the malocclusion.

Swallowing

This is classically divided into the voluntary and involuntary stages. During the voluntary stage of a normal adult swallow, the lips are brought together, the tongue contacts the palate in the region of the rugae, and the teeth are brought lightly together. The bolus is transferred by the tongue to the pharyngeal region where receptors initiate the involuntary stage.

Primary atypical tongue behaviour (endogenous tongue thrust)
Rarely there is an inborn atypical pattern of neuromuscular activity by which the tongue tip retains a more infantile position, and comes forwards to contact the lips during swallowing (an *endogenous* tongue thrust). This can produce both an increase in overjet and a reduction in overbite. Clinically it is difficult to distinguish between the atypical (endogenous) and the *adaptive* tongue behaviour. However, the difference is important since correction of the former is likely to be unstable. The following guidelines may help in recognizing endogenous tongue behaviour:

- The tongue is thrust forwards more forcibly than with adaptive patterns and the amount of circumoral contraction seems to be greater than would have been expected from the degree of lip incompetence.
- The incompleteness of the overbite is greater than is found with adaptive tongue behaviour associated with lip incompetence or a large overjet. Remember that digit-sucking habits or increased anterior skeletal face height may be associated with a similar vertical incisor arrangement.

Other oral tissues

Fraenum

The upper labial fraenum has been implicated in the persistence of a midline diastema (see Chapter 8).

The lower midline labial fraenum may retain its point of attachment high on the gingival margin of the lower incisors, and the pull exerted by this may lead to the formation of a Stillman's cleft. While this, in itself, will not contribute to a malocclusion, from a periodontal point of view the poor prognosis may influence the orthodontic extraction pattern, especially in the adult.

Periodontal and effects of other tissues

It is clear that cellular events within the periodontal ligament and adjacent alveolar bone probably mediate tooth movement (see Chapter 15). The mucosa surrounding the teeth remodels at a much slower rate than the alveolar bone. The supracrestal periodontal fibres have been shown to stretch when a tooth is derotated, and take up to nine months to reorganize fully. This has implications for the length of retention following treatment (see Chapter 25).

Reduction of an overjet using a removal appliance may be hindered by an accumulation of the soft tissues palatal to the upper incisors. Unless provision is made for the soft tissues to build up by judicious trimming of the baseplate, tooth movement can be brought to a halt, and the soft tissues ulcerate and cause pain as they become trapped between the baseplate and the teeth (see Chapter 16).

Mouth breathing

It has been suggested that mouth breathing may influence the skeletal pattern. A major difficulty is in determining exactly what defines 'mouth breathing'. A lips-apart posture does not necessarily signify exclusive breathing through the mouth – the tongue may seal off the oral airway by contact with the palate, and the normal situation of nasal breathing may exist. However, obstruction of the naso-pharyngeal airway by a chronic allergic condition, adenoid hyperplasia or other physical obstruction will result in a downward and forward tongue posture, a lowered mandibular position and a tilted back head posture to permit mouth breathing. If this situation continues for a prolonged period the typical 'adenoid face' may develop. This may be identified as a lips-apart posture, a long face (increased maxillo-mandibular planes angle, with the possibility of an anterior open bite), narrow nostrils, usually a Class II skeletal pattern, with a constricted maxillary arch and upright incisors. There is limited evidence to support the view that removal of the blockage will lead to a resolution of the skeletal and dento-alveolar problems.

It has been proposed that rapid expansion of the maxilla, perhaps with surgical removal of the tonsils and adenoids, may help to correct mouth breathing by increasing the size of the nasal airway. This remains a controversial, if interesting, approach to the correction of this type of problem.

Further reading

Proffit, W.R. (1972). Lingual pressures in the transition from tongue thrust to adult swallowing. *Archives of Oral Biology*, **17**, 555–63.

Proffit, W.R. (1978). Equilibrium theory revisited. *Angle Orthodontist*, **48**, 175–86.

Proffit, W.R. (1993). The aetiology of orthodontic problems. In *Contemporary Orthodontics*, 2nd edn, pp. 130–3. St Louis: Mosby Year Book.

Chapter 6

Development of normal occlusion

Occlusal development may be divided into five stages:

Stage 1. Birth to establishment of deciduous dentition.
Stage 2. Deciduous dentition to early mixed dentition.
Stage 3. Early mixed dentition to late mixed dentition.
Stage 4. Late mixed dentition to permanent dentition.
Stage 5. Permanent dentition.

While these stages form a convenient basis for description, occlusal development should be considered a continuous process that does not cease with the establishment of the full permanent dentition.

Stage 1. Birth to establishment of deciduous dentition

At birth, the maxillary and mandibular gum pads have segmented elevations corresponding to the unerupted deciduous teeth. The elevations for the second deciduous molars are poorly defined at birth and are not properly present until the age of five months. The groove that marks the distal margin of the canine segment continues into the buccal sulcus and is called the 'lateral sulcus'.

The upper arch is horseshoe-shaped and the vault of the palate is very shallow. The alveolar part is separated on its palatal side from the hard palate by a continuous horizontal groove known as the 'dental groove' or 'gingival groove'. The lower arch is U-shaped and the gum pad anteriorly is slightly everted labially.

With the mandible in its physiological rest position the gum pads are apart, with the tongue filling the space between them and projecting against the lips anteriorly, the lower lip forming the principal boundary to the front of the oral cavity. The upper lip appears to be very short at this age.

The gum pads rarely come into occlusion. The maxillary gum pad overlaps the mandibular both buccally and labially, corresponding to the ultimate occlusal relationship of the teeth (Figure 6.1). The gum pads at birth are too small to accommodate the developing incisors, which are crowded and rotated. During the first year of life the gum pads grow rapidly, especially laterally, which permits the incisors to erupt in good alignment, helped by pressure from the tongue and lips.

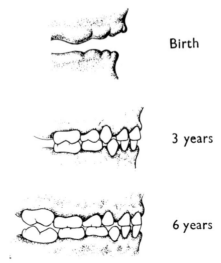

Birth

3 years

6 years

Figure 6.1 Stages in the development of normal occlusion

Neonatal teeth

Occasionally a child is born with teeth already erupted. These are termed neonatal teeth. They are usually present in the lower jaw, are normal teeth from the deciduous series, and have little root development. This, in turn, means that they are often quite mobile; however, there is no indication to remove them unless they are interfering with feeding by causing ulceration of the underside of the tongue, or discomfort to the mother during breast-feeding, or if they are so loose that there is a danger of exfoliation. They should not be confused with gingival cysts of the newborn (Epstein's pearls or Bohn's nodules), which are keratin-filled cysts derived from the dental lamina.

The deciduous dentition (Table 6.1)

Eruption of the lower central incisors begins at about six months of age. It should be recognized that the timing of eruption is very variable and a range of six months on either side of the representative figures given in Table 6.1 is commonplace. Usually by about the age of $2\frac{1}{2}$ years all the deciduous teeth have erupted (Figure 6.1).

Points to notice at $2\frac{1}{2}$ years:

- The incisors are more vertical than their permanent successors and they are often spaced.
- In a normally developing occlusion, there will be spacing distal to the lower canines and mesial to the upper canines (the so-called 'primate spacing').
- In a normally developing occlusion, the distal surfaces of the second deciduous molars should end in line with each other (termed the 'flush terminal plane'). Where the lower deciduous molar is distal to the lower molar (i.e. a Class II molar relationship), it is termed a distal step. Where the lower molar is mesial to the upper molar (i.e. a Class III relationship) it is termed a mesial step.

Table 6.1 Typical ages of eruption and mesiodistal widths of the deciduous teeth

	Time of eruption (months)	*Mesiodistal width* (mm)
Maxillary teeth		
Central incisor	8	6.5
Lateral incisor	9	5.0
Canine	18	6.5
First molar	14	7.0
Second molar	24	8.5
Mandibular teeth		
Central incisor	6	4.0
Lateral incisor	7	4.5
Canine	16	5.5
First molar	12	8.0
Second molar	20	9.5

Notes:
1. Mesiodistal widths vary by up to 20% on either side of the figures given.
2. Calcification of the deciduous teeth begins between 4 and 6 months *in utero*.
3. Root formation is complete between 12 and 18 months after eruption.
4. There is often a difference of a few weeks between tooth eruption on the left and right sides.
5. Usually the lower teeth erupt ahead of their upper counterparts.

Stage 2. Deciduous dentition to early mixed dentition (Table 6.2)

At the age of six years permanent teeth, usually the first molars or lower central incisors start to erupt. As in the case of the deciduous teeth, eruption times and the order of eruption are very variable and a range of 18 months on either side of the figures given in Table 6.2 is not unusual.

Table 6.2 Typical ages of eruption and mesiodistal widths of the permanent teeth

	Time of eruption (years)	*Mesiodistal width* (mm)
Maxillary teeth		
Central incisor	7.5	8.5
Lateral incisor	8.5	6.5
Canine	11.5	8.0
First premolar	10.0	7.0
Second premolar	11.0	6.5
First molar	6.0	10.0
Second molar	12.0	9.5
Mandibular teeth		
Central incisor	6.5	5.5
Lateral incisor	7.5	6.0
Canine	10.0	7.0
First premolar	10.5	7.0
Second premolar	11.0	7.0
First molar	6.0	11.0
Second molar	12.0	10.5

Notes:
1. The figures given both for eruption times and mesiodistal widths commonly vary by up to 20% on either side of the figures given.
2. Calcification dates are variable but the permanent teeth have usually started to calcify as follows: At Birth $\frac{6}{6}$, by 6 months $\frac{13}{123}$, by 2 years $\frac{24}{4}$, by 4 years $\frac{57}{57}$, between 8 and 14 years $\frac{8}{8}$.
3. Root formation is normally completed 2–3 years after eruption.

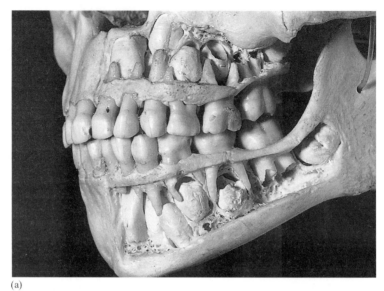

(a)

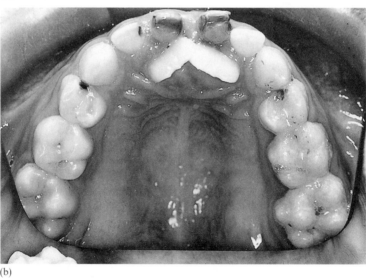

(b)

Figure 6.2 (a) Developmental positions of the permanent incisors. Note that the permanent incisors develop lingual to the roots of the deciduous incisors and that the upper lateral incisors are overlapped by the central incisors and canines. (b) Palatal eruption of permanent upper central incisors. Note retained deciduous predecessors

The permanent incisors

The permanent incisors develop lingual to the roots of the deciduous incisors (Figure 6.2a). Space for these teeth, which are larger than their deciduous predecessors, is provided by:

- Utilization of existing spacing between the deciduous incisors.
- A growth increase in intercanine basal bone width, which takes place during

the eruption of the incisors.
- The upper permanent incisors are more proclined and thus form a larger arch than the deciduous incisors.

Notes
1. If the deciduous incisor root is not resorbed normally, the permanent incisor may be deflected lingually (Figure 6.2b).
2. The upper lateral incisors in their developmental position are overlapped by the central incisors (Figure 6.2a). They escape as the central incisors erupt. However, if there is insufficient growth in arch width they may be trapped in this palatal position.
3. The 'ugly duckling' stage: when the upper incisors erupt they are frequently distally inclined so that there is a median diastema (Figure 6.3). This is due to the incisor roots being crowded mesially by the permanent canine crowns. Additional features that characterize the ugly duckling stage are the large permanent incisors (with their prominent mammelons) in a child-size face; these are darker and less regular than their deciduous predecessors. This natural developmental stage should not be mistaken for a malocclusion and treatment must not be undertaken to close the midline diastema before the permanent canines erupt.
4. There is usually a small growth spurt associated with the eruption of the first permanent molars leading to an increase in face height and a growth in width across the canine region to accommodate the larger permanent incisor teeth (see Chapter 3). This growth in width usually ceases at around the age of 9 years.

The permanent molars

The upper permanent molars develop in the maxillary tuberosity with their occlusal surfaces facing distally and buccally as well as occlusally. Posterior

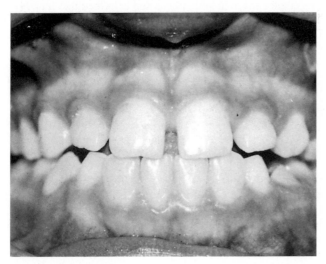

Figure 6.3 The 'ugly duckling' stage

growth in maxillary length is necessary to allow them to rotate forwards and downwards into the line of the arch. The mandibular molars develop under the anterior border of the ascending ramus of the mandible. Growth in mandibular length, which involves resorption on the anterior margin of the ascending ramus, is necessary if the tooth is to have room to erupt.

The permanent molars are guided into position by the distal surfaces of the second deciduous molars. In a normal occlusal relationship the flush terminal plane of the deciduous molars brings the first permanent molars into cusp-to-cusp contact (see also bullet point 3 under 'Stage 1. Birth to establishment of deciduous dentition', on page 50). Asynchronous growth between the maxilla and mandible, and/or premature loss of deciduous molars may contribute to a Class II or Class III molar relationship.

Stage 3. Early mixed dentition to late mixed dentition

After the rapid and dramatic changes that occur during the transition from deciduous to permanent incisors, and the eruption of the first permanent molars, there is a lull in occlusal development for about 12–18 months. The start of the next stage is usually signalled by the eruption of the mandibular canines and maxillary first premolars.

Stage 4. Late mixed dentition to permanent dentition

During this phase the remaining deciduous teeth are shed and replaced by their permanent successors and the second permanent molars erupt.

Leeway space

The discrepancy between the mesiodistal widths of the deciduous molars and the premolars creates space in both arches and is termed the 'leeway space'. The leeway space is greater in the lower arch than the upper arch, and this allows the lower permanent molar to move forwards further than the upper molar and establish a Class I molar relationship; i.e. the mesiobuccal cusp of the maxillary first permanent molar occludes with the mid-buccal groove of the lower first permanent molar. The second permanent molars should be guided directly into occlusion by the distal surfaces of the first permanent molars. See above for descriptions of anomalous molar relationships.

Stage 5. Permanent dentition

The variability of presence and morphology of the third molars means that these teeth are rarely considered in descriptions of occlusion. Angle's classification was based on the relationship of the first molars, a normal or Class I molar relationship described as above. More recently Andrews has described six keys to a normal occlusion, i.e. these are features that are commonly found in non-orthodontic, well-ordered occlusions. They form a basis for identifying deviations from a normal occlusion and a treatment goal for orthodontic correction.

Key I. Molar relationship:

- The distal surface of the distal marginal ridge of the upper first permanent molar contacts and occludes with the mesial surface of the mesial marginal ridge of the lower second molar.
- The mesiobuccal cusp of the upper first permanent molar falls within the groove between the mesial and middle cusps of the lower first permanent molar.
- The mesiolingual cusp of the upper first permanent molar seats in the central fossa of the lower first permanent molar.

Key II. Crown angulation:

The gingival portion of the long axis of each crown is distal to the occlusal portion of that axis, i.e. each tooth crown has a mesiodistal tip and this varies with each tooth.

Key III. Crown inclination:

For upper incisors the gingival portion of the labial surface of the crown is lingual to the incisal portion.

For all other teeth the gingival portion of the labial or buccal surface of the crown is labial or buccal to the incisal/occlusal portion. This is called labiolingual torque.

Key IV. Rotations:

There should be no rotations.

Key V. Contacts:

Provided there are no genuine tooth-size discrepancies, there should be tight contact points.

Key VI. Curve of Spee:

This is measured from incisors to molars and should not exceed a depth of 1.5 mm.

This is a fairly full description of a static occlusal relationship, to which Roth has added some functional goals for occlusion:

- Centric occlusion and centric relation should coincide.
- Occlusal forces should be directed down the long axes of the posterior teeth.
- There should be 0.005 in (0.1270 mm) space between the anterior teeth when in occlusion.
- In lateral and protrusive mandibular movements the canines and incisors disclude the posterior teeth.

He calls this a mutually protective occlusal scheme whereby the posterior teeth protect the anterior teeth in occlusion, and the anterior teeth protect the posterior teeth during mandibular excursions.

While Roth, and other orthodontists, favour mutually protective (also referred to as canine-guided) occlusion as a functional goal, it must be emphasized that there is little scientific evidence to support either canine guidance, or the alternative occlusal philosophy of group function, as the ideal functional occlusion.

Changes in the permanent occlusion

The eruption into occlusion of all the permanent teeth (except the third molars) between the ages of 12 and 14 years does not mark the end of occlusal change.

Incisor crowding
Increasing incisor crowding may be associated with mandibular growth rotations and/or dento-alveolar changes such as reductions in arch width, depth and perimeter. This occurs to a greater extent in males, but is almost ubiquitous and could be considered a normal occlusal developmental feature.

Mesial drift
It has also been suggested that mesial drift of buccal teeth may contribute to this late crowding. Mesial drift is observed when the continuity of the arch is broken by extraction of teeth but the cause is not understood. The following explanations have been offered:

1. It is a natural growth tendency in the human.
2. Crowded teeth, particularly third molars, exert a forward pressure on the other teeth. It should be noted, however, that mesial drift occurs even where third molars are developmentally absent.
3. The anterior component of force: this arises because the upper and lower teeth are slightly mesially inclined. Vertical occlusal loading produces an intrusive force and a small anterior component of force which could be responsible for mesial drift. However, the evidence in support of this theory is insubstantial.

It is disappointing to realize that similar changes in the dental arrangement can occur even following orthodontic treatment. There appear to be no good prognostic indicators of an occlusion which will remain stable in the late teenage years and onwards or one which will deteriorate.

Further reading

Andrews, L.F. (1972). The six keys to normal occlusion. *American Journal of Orthodontics*, **62**, 296–309.

Begg, P.R. (1952). Stone Age man's dentition. With reference to anatomically correct occlusion, the aetiology of occlusion, and a technique for its treatment. *American Journal of Orthodontics*, **40**, 298–312, 373–83, 462–75, 517–31.

Bishara, S.E., Khadivi, P. and Jokobsen, J.R. (1995). Changes in tooth size-arch length relationships from deciduous to the permanent dentition: a longitudinal study. *American Journal of Orthodontics and Dentofacial Orthopedics*, **108**, 607–13.

Moorees, C.F.A., Gron, A.M., Lebret, L.M. *et al.* (1969). Growth studies of the dentition – a review. *American Journal of Orthodontics*, **55**, 600–16.

Roth, R.H. (1976). The maintenance system and occlusal dynamics. *Dental Clinics of North America*, **20**, 761–88.

Sinclair, P.M. and Little, R.M. (1983). Maturation of untreated malocclusions. *American Journal of Orthodontics*, **83**, 114–23.

Chapter 7

Malocclusion

A malocclusion is defined as an irregularity of the teeth or a malrelationship of the dental arches beyond the accepted range of normal. Thus malocclusions are for the most part variations around the normal and are a representation of biological variability. Biological variation is expressed elsewhere in the body but minor irregularities are more readily noticed and recorded in the dentition and so have attracted greater attention with an associated demand for treatment. The majority of malocclusions are primarily of hereditary causation although environmental factors, for example the unplanned extraction of teeth, may also contribute.

There is evidence that the prevalence of malocclusion is increasing, particularly in developed communities. This increase may, in part, reflect an underlying evolutionary trend towards shorter jaws and fewer teeth, but it is more probably largely the result of an increase in the genetic variability of these populations brought about by intermixture of racial groups. It has been proposed by Begg that one reason for the increase in the prevalence of crowding is that there is now little approximal or occlusal attrition of the teeth. In primitive people living on a coarse diet an appreciable reduction in the mesiodistal widths of erupted teeth occurs due to attrition. This loss of tooth substance, which can amount to several millimetres in each quadrant, would reduce a tendency to crowding. Unfortunately, there is little solid evidence to support this view.

Malocclusions may be associated with one or more of the following:

- malposition of individual teeth
- malrelationship of the dental arches.

Malocclusion of individual teeth

A tooth may occupy a position other than normal by being:

1. *Tipped* – the tooth apex is normally placed but the crown is incorrectly positioned. Teeth may be tipped laterally (termed angulation) or may be tipped labiopalatally (termed inclination).
2. *Displaced* – both apex and crown are incorrectly positioned.
3. *Rotated* – the tooth is rotated around its long axis.
4. *In infraocclusion* – the tooth has not reached the occlusal level.
5. *In supraocclusion* – the tooth has erupted past the occlusal level.

6. *Transposed* – two teeth have reversed their positions; an example of this might be an upper canine and first premolar.

Teeth that are tilted or displaced are described according to the direction of the malposition: for example, an incisor may be labially inclined (or proclined), lingually inclined (or retroclined), mesially angulated, or distally angulated. Similar terms may be applied to displacements. Rotations are probably best described by the approximal surface that is furthest from the line of the arch and the direction it faces. As an example, a rotated upper incisor is described as mesiolabially rotated if the mesial aspect is out of the line of the arch, whilst a similar rotation would be described as distopalatal if the distal aspect was palatally positioned.

There are two terms commonly used to describe the relationship of upper to lower incisors:

The overjet is defined as the horizontal overlap of the incisors. Usually the upper and lower incisors are in contact and the overlap reflects the thickness of the upper incisor edge – usually 2 to 3 mm. When the lower incisors are ahead of the uppers this is termed a negative or reverse overjet.

The overbite is defined as the vertical overlap of the incisors. Usually the lower incisor edge is in contact with the middle of the palatal surface of the upper incisor; this area is called the cingulum. Normally the overbite is about 2 mm. On occasions it may be significantly reduced until there is a vertical gap between the tooth edges: this is called an 'anterior openbite'. If the overbite is increased this may lead to a 'deep overbite', which may, on occasion, be 'complete' to the palate.

Malrelationship of the dental arches

Malrelationships of the arches may occur in any of the three planes of space: antero-posterior, vertical or transverse. The aetiology and treatment of vertical and transverse malrelationships are dealt with in Chapter 10. The classifications of malocclusion described in this text are based on antero-posterior relationships as described below. The aetiology and treatment of these malrelationships are dealt with in Chapters 11–14.

Classification of malocclusion

For convenience of description, it is useful to have some classification that will divide up the wide range of malocclusions into a small number of groups. Many classifications have been proposed but the one that is universally recognized is Angle's classification, which is based, in the first instance, on the arch relationship in the sagittal plane. The key relationship in Angle's classification is that of the first permanent molars: it is suggested that in normal occlusions, the anterior buccal groove of the lower first permanent molar should occlude with the anterior buccal cusp of the upper first permanent molar (see Figure 1.1). If the first molars have drifted, allowance must be made for this before the occlusion is classified. In functional terms, a Class I molar relationship is better defined

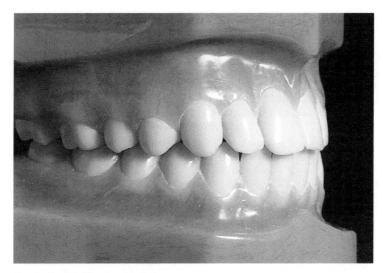

Figure 7.1 An Angle's Class I malocclusion

by the position of the upper distobuccal cusp of the first molar interdigitating and contacting the embrasure between the distobuccal cusp of the lower first molar and mesiobuccal cusp of the lower second molar.

Angle's classification

Class I. Malocclusions in which the lower first permanent molar is within one half-cusp width of its correct relationship to the upper first permanent molar (Figure 7.1). This arch relationship is sometimes known as 'neutro-occlusion'.

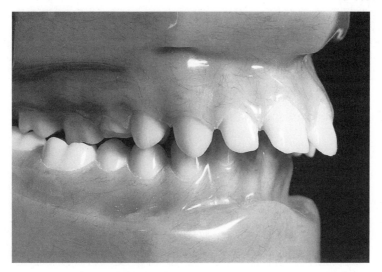

Figure 7.2 An Angle's Class II Division 1 malocclusion

Class II. The lower arch is at least one-half cusp width posterior to the correct relationship with the upper arch, judged by the first molar relationship (Figures 5.3 and 7.2). This arch relationship is sometimes known as 'disto-occlusion'.

Class II may be further subdivided according to the inclination of the upper central incisors:

> **Division 1.** The upper central incisors are proclined or of average inclination with an increase in the overjet (Figure 7.2).
>
> **Division 2.** The upper central incisors are retroclined (Figure 7.3), being less than 105° to the maxillary plane. The overjet is usually of an average size but may be a little increased. Sometimes the upper lateral incisors are proclined, mesially inclined and mesiolabially rotated.

Class III. The lower arch is at least one-half cusp width too far forward in relation to the upper arch, judged by the first permanent molar relationship. This arch relationship is sometimes known as 'mesio-occlusion'.

A number of problems may be encountered when attempting to classify a particular malocclusion according to Angle's method.

1. The first permanent molars may have been extracted or they may have drifted following early loss of deciduous molar teeth (Figure 7.4). Where the first molars have drifted forwards as a result of early loss, due allowance should be made before classification. This is not always simple and it is well worthwhile looking at the general features of the occlusion and, in particular, at the permanent canine relationship. The upper permanent canine should occlude into the embrasure between the lower canine and first premolar. This relationship should match the first permanent molar relationship: in Class II cases the embrasure between the lower canine and first premolar will be distal to the cusp of the upper canine; in Class III cases, it will be too far forwards. In general, if the molar and canine relationship match one another, the classification can be affirmed with reasonable confidence; but if they do

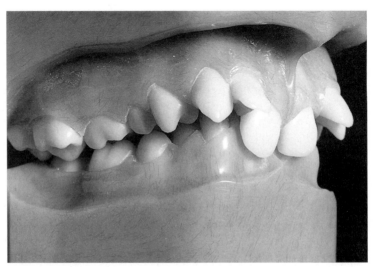

Figure 7.3 An Angle's Class II Division 2 malocclusion

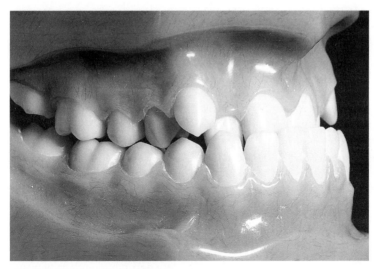

Figure 7.4 An Angle's Class III malocclusion

not, care must be taken and classification may have to be undertaken on the general features of the occlusion.
2. The occlusion may differ between sides. Angle allowed for this by describing subdivisions of Class II and Class III where one side was in a normal relationship. However, it is probably more useful to classify the occlusion according to its general features.
3. It can be difficult to know where to draw the dividing line between Class I and the other classes. Here again, the final decision must rest on the general features of the occlusion. It is often helpful to look also to the position of the upper distobuccal cusp of the first permanent molar. In a Class I relationship with good function, this normally occludes to the embrasure between the lower first and second permanent molars.

Angle considered that the first permanent molars had constant developmental relationships to their respective jaws so that, by classifying the occlusion, the skeletal pattern could also be assessed. It must be emphasized that this assumption is not correct and that the developmental positions of the teeth on the jaws may vary. Thus the occlusal and skeletal classifications may not necessarily coincide. It is usually helpful to classify the skeletal, molar and incisor relationships separately since their classifications do not always coincide.

Incisor classification

The incisor relationship does not always match the buccal segment relationship. Since much of orthodontic treatment is focused on the correction of incisor malrelationships, it is helpful to have a classification of incisor relationships (Figure 7.5). The terms used are the same but this is not Angle's classification, although it is a derivation. In clinical practice the incisor classification is usually found to be more useful than Angle's classification.

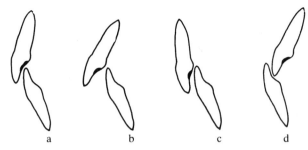

Figure 7.5 Incisor classification: (a) Class I; (b) Class II Division 1; (c) Class II Division 2; (d) Class III

Class I. The lower incisor edges occlude with or lie immediately below the cingulum plateau (middle part of the palatal surface) of the upper central incisors (Figure 7.5a).

Class II. The lower incisor edges lie posterior to the cingulum plateau of the upper incisors.
    There are two divisions to Class II malocclusion:
    Division 1. The upper central incisors are proclined or of average inclination, with an increased overjet (Figure 7.5b).
    Division 2. The upper central incisors are retroclined (less than 105° to the maxillary plane). The overjet is usually of an average size but may be increased (Figure 7.5c).

Class III. The lower incisor edges lie anterior to the cingulum plateau of the upper incisors (Figure 7.5d). The overjet may be either reduced or reversed.

Aetiology of malocclusion

For the convenience of this discussion, the causes of malocclusion can broadly be divided into general factors and local factors.
    General factors are discussed in detail in the relevant chapters and include variations in skeletal relationship (Chapter 3), disproportion between tooth and arch size that may result in either crowding or spacing (Chapter 9) and soft tissue factors (Chapter 5).
    Malocclusions may also be associated with a number of genetic and developmental disorders; examples of this might include Down's syndrome (mongolism), hypothyroidism (cretinism), cleidocranial dysostosis and many other relatively uncommon syndromes. To maintain the brevity of the current text these will not be discussed further here. However, due to the dental importance and comparative frequency of cleft lip and palate, this condition is discussed further in Chapter 23.
    Local factors are essentially habits and anomalies in the number, form and developmental positions of the teeth. In spite of their classification as local factors, their effects may be quite extensive. Local factors may coexist with one another and with any of the general factors mentioned above.

Further reading

Angle, E.H. (1899). Classification of malocclusion. *Dental Cosmos*, **41**, 248–64.

Begg, P.R. (1954). Stone Age man's dentition. *American Journal of Orthodontics*, **40**, 298–312.

British Standards Institute (1983). *Glossary of Dental Terms* (BS 4492). London: BSI.

Gravely, J.F. and Johnston, D.B. (1974). Angle's classification of malocclusion: an assessment of reliability. *British Journal of Orthodontics*, **61**, 286–94.

Chapter 8

Aetiology and management of the abnormally developing occlusion: interceptive orthodontics

Unfortunately most occlusions do not develop in the normal manner described earlier in Chapter 6. Indeed in excess of 60% of children have a variation from normal development leading to a malocclusion. To understand fully the impact of abnormal development and hence the consideration of timing of correction it is relevant to develop a knowledge of why the occlusion may develop in an abnormal way. It is important to understand that the cause of malocclusion involves a complex interaction of genetic factors (those inherited from a certain specific or mixed genetic pool) and environmental factors, where the genetic predisposition to a type of occlusal development can be modified by factors in the surrounding tissues and spaces. Malocclusion can be caused by variation in the size of the jaws (skeletal factors) or a variation in the relationship of the dentition to the jaw size (arch length discrepancies). In addition local environmental factors can affect one particular area of the dentition to create a malocclusion.

Skeletal factors

As the alveolus and the basal bones of the maxilla and mandible support the teeth, any deviation from ideal growth and development can be reflected in a malrelationship of the teeth. It is also important to remember that the face is a three-dimensional structure so that any variation from normal development can occur in each plane or in a combination of any of the three planes.

Sagittal. Here there is a difference in the relationship of the maxilla and the mandible in the anterior-posterior plane. This can be due to a combination of factors:

- the maxilla is too large or small opposite a normal-sized mandible
- the mandible is too large or small opposite a normal-sized maxilla
- there is some variation in size of both the upper and lower jaws in the opposite direction.

If the magnitude of variation is sufficiently large the teeth, as they erupt, cannot *compensate* for the difference. One usually then sees a variation in the incisor relationship that reflects some or all of the sagittal skeletal discrepancy (see Figures 12.1 and 14.1).

Vertical. Here there is a difference in the relationship of the upper face height (i.e. the maxilla) and the lower face height (i.e. the mandible). In addition, sometimes there can be a difference between the vertical development of the total anterior face height and the total posterior face height (see Chapter 3). Again, if this malrelationship is sufficiently severe it can be reflected in a variation in the position of the incisor teeth, which might be anything from an *anterior open bite* to a *deep overbite*. The latter may, occasionally, result in trauma to the soft tissues, to the gingivae either labial to the lower labial segment or palatal to the upper incisors (Figure 8.1).

Transverse. Here there is a difference in the lateral relationship of the maxilla and the mandible. The most common causes of this are when the maxillary dentition is narrow and opposed by a normal-sized mandible. Alternatively it may be seen when a normal-sized maxilla is opposed by a wider region of the mandible. This malrelationship is manifest clinically by the presence of a buccal crossbite. This can either be unilateral (one-sided) or bilateral (both sides). Less frequent is the condition of a lingual crossbite ('scissors bite'). Here the upper teeth in the buccal segment occlude to the outside of the mandibular dentition (Figure 8.2).

This transverse malrelationship of the dental bases is an important cause of malocclusion in the developing dentition. Where a transverse malrelationship of the bases exists then occasionally the mandible on its arc of closure may bring the teeth into premature contact with one or more maxillary teeth. This, in turn, may cause the mandible to be displaced from its normal path of closure to a position of maximum occlusion, which is not consistent with the centric relation of the condyle in the glenoid fossa. This has been implicated as a cause of craniomandibular dysfunction (or temporomandibular pain dysfunction syndrome), although the evidence remains controversial. However, this occlusal problem is amenable to early orthodontic correction, and expansion of the maxilla is possible in the mixed dentition to eliminate this displacement (Figure 8.3). This can be achieved with either slow expansion (using a removable appliance or a fixed quadhelix) or rapid expansion (using a palatal expander to

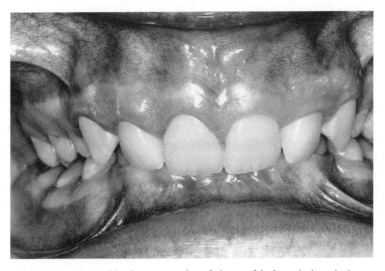

Figure 8.1 Deep overbite resulting in trauma to the soft tissues of the lower incisor gingivae

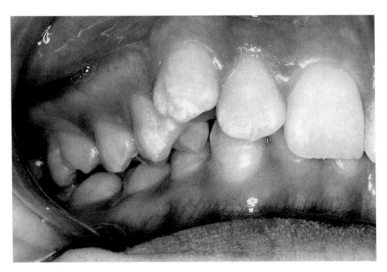

Figure 8.2 Lingual crossbite or scissors bite

achieve orthopaedic separation of the intermaxillary suture, which is not completely fused until the late teenage years.

Arch length discrepancy

This may present as a malocclusion where there is variation between the size of the dental arches and the size, or position, of the erupting dentition.

The dentition develops within the confines of the basal bones. On eruption of the teeth there may be insufficient space to accommodate the dentition without irregularity. This is then manifest as crowding. As discussed in Chapters 3 and 6, one can expect some change in arch dimension with growth. However, after the age of about 9–10 years very little change in arch perimeter size occurs. Any need to obtain space to accommodate arch length discrepancy requires careful consideration.

Crowding

When the size of the dentition is greater than the space available to accommodate the teeth in good general alignment then crowding may be said to occur. In the early mixed dentition some degree of crowding is normal and up to the age of 8–9 years one can expect to see some spontaneous improvement in incisor alignment. After this age spontaneous alignment is unlikely. Occasionally, if there is far too little space for the developing maxillary incisors then a lateral incisor may be deflected palatally resulting in a localized single tooth in crossbite with insufficient space.

Crowding in the labial segments in the mixed dentition has been the subject of much debate in the orthodontic literature. Anecdotally there has been a traditionally held belief that obtaining alignment of the labial segments at an

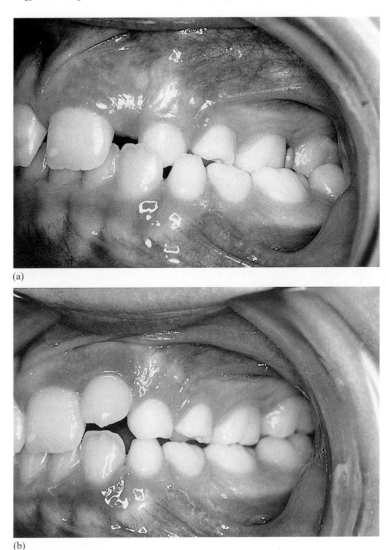

(a)

(b)

Figure 8.3 (a) Buccal crossbite associated with a mandibular displacement. (b) Following treatment with a quadhelix for upper arch expansion

early age may enhance the stability of the resulting alignment. To achieve this result Kjelleren introduced the concept of 'serial extraction' in 1948.

Serial extraction
In this therapeutic intervention it is suggested that, in Class I malocclusions with developing incisor crowding, extraction of deciduous teeth, initially the decid-uous canines followed by first deciduous molars may be advantageous. This is intended to facilitate the alignment of the teeth of the labial segments and promote the eruption of the first premolars before the permanent canines. These events, combined with the increasing severity of the crowding in the buccal

segments, are said to lead to favourable conditions for extraction of the first premolars and subsequent spontaneous alignment of the permanent canines.

Such an approach might be considered initially at 7–8 years of age with loss of deciduous canines, then followed with almost yearly interventions for extraction of first deciduous molars (when roots of the first premolars, bicuspids, are half formed) and then finally the first premolars (bicuspids) (see Chapter 9).

The benefits of such an approach have to be balanced against the possible risks associated with three episodes of exodontia and the reliability of a predicted outcome. Little hard evidence exists, outside case reports, as to the value of such an approach in reducing overall treatment time or complexity, or in enhancing stability.

Displaced erupting incisor

In some circumstances early correction of a maxillary incisor that has erupted into a lingually displaced position can produce significant and sustainable benefit to the occlusion. This might involve the early balanced removal of deciduous canines to gain sufficient space. Simple removable appliance therapy can be provided, if a sufficient space exists or can be created, to correct the reverse overjet on the tooth. Care must be taken in the assessment of the condition that no generalized maxillary transverse constriction exists and that any posterior crossbite should be corrected if present.

Spacing

More rarely one sees the condition where the arch perimeter is greater than the combined mesiodistal widths of the dentition even when all the teeth are present. Under such circumstances it is likely that generalized spacing will be evident between the teeth. This is generally refractory to orthodontic correction and indeed a spaced dentition is less susceptible to caries than one with intact contact points or crowding! If aesthetics are compromised a joint approach involving a combined restorative orthodontic approach may be indicated.

Curve of Spee

To obtain ideal occlusal goals it is desirable during orthodontic treatment to produce a flat occlusal plane. However, if the occlusal plane has a significant curve of Spee an increase in arch length will be required to accommodate the flattening of this curve. Fixed appliance mechanics to flatten a curve of Spee will cause an increase in arch length and therefore this effect must be considered during the assessment of space requirements during treatment planning.

Incisor inclination

In certain rare circumstances it is also considered necessary to alter the labial segment inclination. As an example, any significant proclination of the lower incisors will adversely influence the arch length. This might occur in the case of bimaxillary proclination where the incisors might be required to be retracted for facial aesthetics. In this situation, not only will space be required for relief of crowding and to level the curve of Spee but also additional space will be needed to accommodate this labial segment retraction.

Local factors

The issues of skeletal and arch length discrepancy most usually affect the whole malocclusion. However, many of the variations from ideal may be confined to just one part of the occlusion. These are often referred to as local factors and can be a common cause of malocclusion.

Variation in tooth number

Hypodontia
This means the congenital absence of teeth. It can affect both the deciduous and permanent dentitions but is more common in the permanent dentition. Brook in 1974 reported a prevalence of 4.4%, with the teeth most commonly absent (excluding third molars) being second premolars, maxillary lateral incisors and mandibular incisors. However, it is possible to have any tooth congenitally absent and any combination may occur. The management of hypodontia is complicated and requires comprehensive assessment and treatment planning. McNeill and Joondeph, in 1973, suggested that the primary factor to consider is the malocclusion (e.g. the degree of crowding). After this the secondary factor to consider is the morphology of the local standing teeth, for example the size, shape and colour of cuspids if they were to be advanced to replace missing lateral incisors. It is also important to consider and plan the fate of deciduous teeth retained because of congenital absence of the succadaneous tooth. Loss of such a tooth at the correct time may favourably influence spontaneous space closure and eliminate or reduce active appliance therapy.

Hyperdontia
In hyperdontia a person may develop teeth in addition to the normal number of teeth expected. These are commonly called supernumerary teeth and again can occur anywhere in the mouth. They have a prevalence of approximately 2% in the permanent dentition and most commonly they occur in the anterior region of the maxilla where they are referred to as mesiodens. If they appear similar in morphology to the teeth near where they are located they are referred to as supplemental teeth. Supernumerary teeth can cause failure of eruption or displacement of the adjacent teeth. Early detection and removal of supernumerary teeth usually results in a high chance of spontaneous eruption of delayed teeth, providing sufficient space is available. In the event that the affected permanent tooth fails to erupt a direct attachment and gold chain is often provided to facilitate orthodontic traction to the unerupted tooth (Figure 8.4; also see Chapter 20).

Variation in tooth form

Megadontia
Teeth that are larger than usual can cause difficulties in orthodontic treatment planning. These teeth often have pulp chambers in proportion to the tooth.

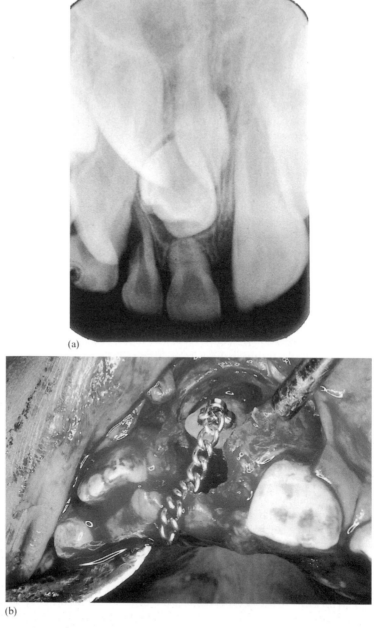

(a)

(b)

Figure 8.4 (a) Unerupted central incisors with supernumerary teeth. (b) Supernumerary teeth removed and gold chain and orthodontic attachment bonded to the unerupted teeth to facilitate traction if spontaneous eruption fails to occur

Seldom can they be easily reduced to the correct size without compromising their vitality, and often their loss as part of an extraction pattern to relieve crowding is indicated.

Microdontia

Occasionally a patient presents with small teeth, often associated with one particular tooth type and most commonly the maxillary lateral incisor. These are often referred to as 'peg laterals' and, again, their long-term viability should be assessed as part of an overall orthodontic treatment plan. Their role as a predictor of position of the maxillary cuspid remains controversial but it appears that missing or small maxillary lateral incisors could be associated with ectopic (usually palatal) eruption of these teeth.

Invaginations

Some patients present with an abnormality of the crown of a tooth. In particular this is found in maxillary lateral incisors where a reversal of the normal layers and an 'invagination' of the enamel structure disrupt the normal arrangement of the dental hard tissues. This can present as mild, as in 'dens-in-dente', or more severe, as an invaginated odontome (Figure 8.5). The management depends on the degree of deformity and the requirements of the overall malocclusion.

Damage due to trauma

Inevitably some children suffer trauma to the deciduous dentition. Trauma to the upper labial segment can result in the deformity of the permanent teeth. This can vary from enamel hypoplasia to severe crown–root dilaceration (Figure 8.6). The management depends on the severity and direction of the dilaceration, but severe deformities are unlikely to be accommodated successfully due to the width of the alveolar process.

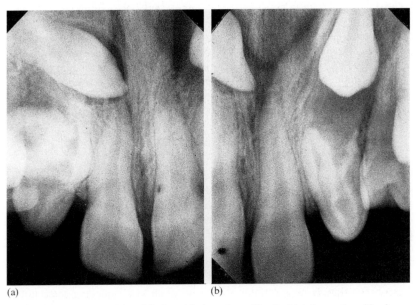

(a)   (b)

Figure 8.5 (a, b) Abnormalities of the lateral incisors due to disturbed development resulting in invaginations or dens-in-dente

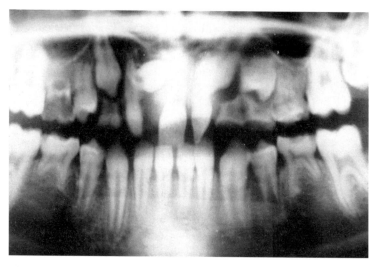

Figure 8.6 Trauma to a deciduous incisor has led to severe crown–root dilaceration of the permanent successor. Also note other associated anomalies: peg laterals, missing teeth and ectopic permanent caries

Variation in tooth position or eruption

Submerged deciduous teeth

This condition occurs when a deciduous tooth appears to lie beneath the occlusal plane of adjacent teeth. It is not uncommon to find the permanent tooth congenitally absent, although it can occur in the presence of a successor. It is believed that the deciduous tooth undergoes ankylosis to the surrounding alveolar bone and fails to 'erupt' and keep pace with the surrounding dentition. A more appropriate term would be infraocclusion. The vast majority of these teeth exfoliate normally as the resorptive phase of the normal eruption process releases the ankylosis. However, it is important to monitor submerging teeth since the 'tipping over' of the adjacent teeth may prevent spontaneous correction and exfoliation of the submerged teeth from occurring. For this reason extraction of the submerged teeth once they go below the contact point of adjacent teeth should be considered.

Premature loss of deciduous teeth

In general terms premature loss of deciduous teeth results in further loss of space for permanent successors and an increase in crowding. In some cases, such as serial extraction, this is a therapeutic decision. In other cases space loss may not be required and space maintenance should be considered, although if teeth are lost prematurely due to caries the oral environment may not be conducive to long-term appliance wear. Sometimes, particularly if there is premature loss of a deciduous canine or first deciduous molar from one side of an arch, the dental centre line may shift towards the side with the tooth loss. In these circumstances consideration should be given to a balancing extraction of the contralateral tooth to minimize the impact of a centre line shift provided this can be accomplished easily and without unnecessary stress to the patient. It is hardly ever necessary to compensate between arches for the loss of deciduous teeth.

Unplanned loss of permanent teeth

First permanent molars
Unfortunately patients with carious first permanent molar teeth still present at the dentist's surgery. In the young patient, where the quality of the first permanent molars raises concern in the mixed dentition, consideration should be given to incorporating them in an extraction pattern if so required. It is considered that an ideal time for their extraction is approximately at 10 years of age or more precisely just as the bifurcation of the second permanent molar begins to form. However, a comprehensive orthodontic treatment plan for each patient should be made. This should include consideration of not only dental development but also presence of other permanent teeth, degree and site of potential crowding, overall space requirements of the malocclusion and the need to extract the contralateral or contravertical first permanent molars. Indeed, patients with such poor quality teeth may not be good candidates for extensive orthodontic therapy.

Ectopic eruption of permanent teeth

Impacted first permanent molars
In some early mixed dentition malocclusions the erupting first permanent molar has insufficient space. This may lead to impaction of the permanent molar into the distal surface of the deciduous second molar. In severe cases the second molar undergoes root resorption and this can result in early exfoliation and space loss. In the milder case the impaction can lead to caries in the mesial surface of the first permanent molar, and if the impaction is significant, consideration should be given to moving the molar distally to release the impaction. It is likely to be an early indication of crowding.

Maxillary cuspid eruption
The maxillary cuspid has the furthest of all the permanent teeth to travel on its path of eruption into the mouth. Therefore, it is not surprising that it is the tooth most likely to exhibit ectopic eruption. Ectopic positioning of the canine occurs in approximately 3% of patients and, of these, over three-quarters are palatally displaced. Some sources suggest that up to 50% of palatally displaced canines are associated with small or congenitally absent lateral incisors. This has led to speculation that a lack of guidance from the root of the lateral incisor could be responsible for the malpositioning. Other authors suggest that there may be a genetic predisposition to the condition. Certainly, early detection of this problem should be a priority for the dental practitioner.

Note: *If the canine is not palpable in the buccal sulcus (just distal to the root of the lateral incisor) by 10 years of age an appropriate radiograph should be taken to assess whether the deciduous tooth is undergoing resorption.*

If this is not the case further films should be taken to localize the permanent canine. If the canine is becoming palatally displaced, extraction of the deciduous canine should be considered. As an interceptive measure extraction of the deciduous tooth has been shown to produce in excess of 70% improvement of the malpositioned canine provided sufficient space is available (Ericson and Kurol, 1988). Failure to diagnose ectopically erupting permanent teeth can mean that a vital opportunity to intercept a developing problem is missed, and may lead to damage of other teeth in the labial segment by root resorption (Figure 8.7).

Transpositions
The developmental position of tooth crypts can occasionally be switched around and in such cases the sequence of teeth within the arch can be reversed. When this occurs between the maxillary cuspid and the first bicuspid it has been suggested that there is a strong genetic basis for its aetiology. Management of such transpositions requires detailed assessment of the malocclusion and an understanding of the requirement and timing of exodontia.

Secondary retention of permanent molars
This rare condition occurs when permanent molar teeth fail to erupt or, consequent upon their eruption, begin to infraocclude. The suggested aetiology is ankylosis but the cause of the ankylosis remains unclear. There is often a stunted dilacerated root pattern on affected molars. These are refractory to orthodontic traction and their removal, as part of an overall treatment plan, should be considered (Figure 8.8).

Soft tissues

Tongue position
The swallowing pattern of a growing child matures in a similar manner to most of the somatic functions of the body. The so-called infantile swallow usually alters as the dentition and feeding habits mature. It has been suggested that in some individuals there is a persistence of the infantile swallow into maturity. This has been labelled an 'endogenous tongue thrust' and if present interposes itself between the teeth on swallowing leading to an increase in overjet and possibly an anterior open bite or reduced overbite. Before reaching the diagnosis of endogenous tongue thrust one must be careful to seek another explanation for the incisor abnormality. The endogenous tongue thrust, if it does occur, is rare. Some authors estimate the incidence at 3.1% of the population. However, its relevance is considerable since any treatment undertaken may well relapse if the positions of the teeth in the labial segment are positioned where such soft tissue pressure would adversely influence them. Most cases in which the tongue is interposed between the teeth in function are due to the need to complete an anterior oral seal during swallowing and are an adaptation to the positioning of the incisor segments. This adaptive tongue thrust will not persist once the incisor abnormality has been corrected.

It is not uncommon in cases of increased overjet that the overjet magnitude is greater than the underlying skeletal discrepancy between the mandible and the maxilla. In such cases the soft tissue position and function often act to increase the severity of the overjet. Moreover, the lower lip often lies behind the upper incisors at rest and during function to obtain an anterior oral seal. This so-called 'lip trap' may exacerbate the proclination of the upper incisors to worsen the overjet relationship. It has also been suggested that excessive function of the

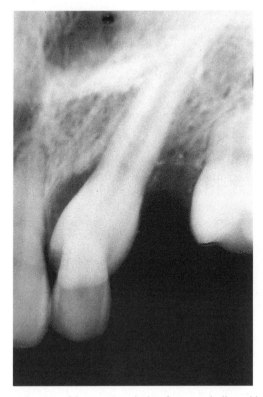

Figure 8.7 Damage to the roots of the permanent incisor from ectopically positioned permanent canine tooth

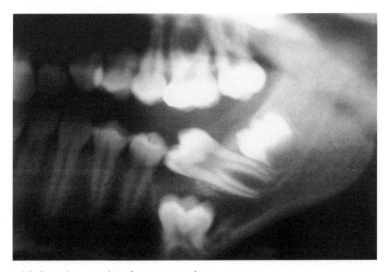

Figure 8.8 Secondary retention of permanent molar

lower lip, often called a 'straplike' lower lip, can lead to excessive retroclination of the lower labial segment in some cases.

Fraenal attachment

The presence of fraenal attachments to the alveolar gingival margin is a normal appearance of the spaced deciduous dentition. With normal development of the alveolar process the fraenal attachment usually migrates apically. The labial fraenae of the lower incisor region occasionally retains a high attachment. In such cases, and particularly where there may be a bony dehiscence on the labial aspect of a tooth, disruption of the integrity of the gingival margin and recession may occur.

In the maxillary dentition it is not uncommon to see the persistence of a low fraenal attachment and a diastema between the central incisors. In fact a diastema here in the mixed dentition is a normal appearance and most commonly this resolves spontaneously on the eruption of the permanent cuspids. Occasionally this persists and it is an easy assumption to make that the frenum is aetiological in the presence of a continued diastema. In such circumstances should treatment for the spacing be provided and the fraenal attachment surgically relieved we may reasonably expect the stability of such a space closure to be enhanced. In fact the evidence that fraenectomy enhances the stability of diastema closure is very limited. Indeed, there is a strong argument that prolonged retention may be a preferred option to the surgical procedure if stability of the diastema closure is the main concern. Sometimes the appearance of a fleshy fraenum is, in itself, sufficient indication for surgical treatment.

Habits

It is known from our understanding of the soft tissue environment surrounding the teeth that they lie in a zone of equilibrium between the balancing forces of these soft tissues. The perioral muscles, the tongue and the periodontal ligament all act both at rest and in function to retain the stable position of the teeth. If any of these forces change, for example loss of periodontal support, or if another force acts for sufficient time and magnitude, the teeth can be influenced to move to a different position. It has been shown that any force acting on the dentition needs to be present for approximately six hours to influence the tooth position. Digit-sucking habits are perhaps the most common example of this influence. A usual presentation of a thumb- or finger-sucking habit in the mixed dentition is evidenced by the presence of a reduced or incomplete overbite, often asymmetrical, proclined upper incisors and/or retroclined lower incisors, and not uncommonly due to increased activity of the buccinator muscle, the presence of a unilateral crossbite. If the habit is broken early many of the presenting signs are reversible. The presence of the crossbite, however, is the least likely to spontaneously resolve and active treatment involving maxillary arch expansion is usually indicated.

Pathology

Syndromes and cleft lip and palate

Major disruption to development in the first trimester of pregnancy can result in severe disturbance in the growth and development of the oro-facial region.

These are produced by a complex interaction of genetic and environmental factors and are more fully described in Chapter 23.

Growth deformity due to trauma

In some children damage due to trauma can extend further than just the teeth. A number of children will suffer damage to the condyles of the mandible following trauma, often due to a minor fall as a 'toddler'. Most of these will resolve without consequence. Lund, in 1974, estimated that 75% of such children do not suffer any disturbance of condylar function on the affected side. In some cases a 'functional ankylosis' can occur. This can have marked effects on the growth of the mandible on the affected side, and complex treatment may be required to restore normal growth and development.

Other pathological processes can affect the developing occlusion but these are fortunately rare. Careful clinical and radiological examination will detect early deviations from normal development and indicate the need for special investigations. Treatment of such cases often involves interdisciplinary team working.

Conclusions

It can be seen that the majority of children will develop a malocclusion. The role of the dental practitioner is to detect early any deviation from normal and consider when, and in what manner, that deviation might require treatment. As can be seen, a thorough knowledge of normal development and continued evaluation of the patient's progress against normal landmarks is required. A careful consideration of interceptive treatments can prevent a number of conditions from progressing to a position where a more complicated treatment might become necessary.

Further reading

Brook, A. (1974). Dental anomalies of number, form and size; their prevalence in UK children. *Journal of the International Association of Dentistry for Children*, **5**, 37–53.

Ericson, S. and Kurol, J. (1988). Early treatment of palatally erupting maxillary canines by extraction of primary canines. *European Journal of Orthodontics*, **10**, 283–9.

Foster, T.D. and Day, A.J.W. (1974). A survey of malocclusion and the need for orthodontic treatment in a Shropshire school population. *British Journal of Orthodontics*, **1**, 73–8.

Kjelleren, B. (1948). Serial extraction as a corrective procedure in dental orthopaedic therapy. *European Orthodontic Society Transactions*, **1**, 37–53.

Lund, K. (1974). Mandibular growth and remodelling process after mandibular fractures. *Acta Odontica Scandinavica*, **32**, (Suppl. 64).

McNeill, R.W. and Joondeph, D.R. (1973). Congenitally missing or absent maxillary lateral incisors; treatment planning considerations. *Angle Orthodontist*, **43**, 24–9.

Chapter 9

Tooth–arch disproportion

Disproportion between tooth size and arch size is common. It is usually manifest as crowding but occasionally there is generalized spacing. Tooth size is under direct genetic control whilst the size of the dental arches depends on skeletal base size and on the soft tissue morphology and activity: as such the dental arch is under the influence of both environmental and genetic factors. This disparity in the factors influencing tooth and arch size goes some way to explaining the tendency to crowding.

Spacing

This is best accepted unless it gives an unsightly appearance in the upper labial segment. In this region, the spacing may be concentrated in the midline as a median diastema. It is sometimes possible to obtain an acceptable result by moving the upper central incisors together, distributing the space mesial and distal to the lateral incisors prior to a build-up in width of these teeth using composite additions or, alternatively, composite or porcelain veneers. A frae-nectomy (Chapter 20) may then be performed to facilitate complete closure; in addition this will help to stabilize the result. When a patient first presents with a median diastema it is important to determine if there is a family history: in such a situation there is usually a strong tendency towards at least a partial relapse, which appears to be determined by the inherited tooth size. A build-up in the width of the relevant incisors with composite or a porcelain veneer can often be of assistance in such cases since it might avoid the need for long-term fixed retention. Sometimes, if the crowns of the lateral incisors are diminutive and contributing to the local spacing, these may be built up in a similar way.

Where spacing is more generalized and if treatment is indicated, appliances may be used to concentrate the spacing in the buccal segments. Some form of prosthesis (preferably a bridge) will then be required both for aesthetic reasons and to assist in preventing relapse.

Crowding

Crowding is common and any teeth may be involved: the incisors and canines if the arch is narrow or short; the molars where the arch is short (see Figure 9.1);

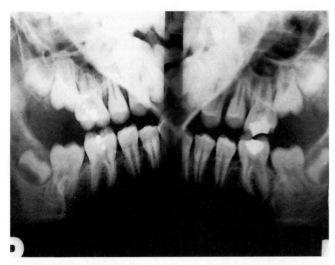

Figure 9.1 Crowding in the upper and lower molar regions. The upper molars are 'stacked'. The lower third molars will be impacted

the premolars and canines if there has been drift of teeth following early loss of deciduous molars (see Chapter 8).

In general, it is not possible to produce a stable increase in arch size by labial movement of incisors or lateral expansion of buccal segments. Provided that the skeletal bases are long and the molars are not crowded, small amounts of space can sometimes be gained by distal movement of buccal segments using extra-oral traction (see Chapter 17). However, if appreciable amounts of space are required to relieve crowding, extractions are required. Clearly, the poor condition or abnormal form of any teeth will influence the choice of extraction. However, in the following discussion it will be assumed, unless explicitly stated otherwise, that all permanent teeth are present and sound. To an extent, whether or not an active appliance is to be employed and the type of appliance also will dictate the choice of extraction. As an example, where crowding of the arches is moderate with little overjet or overbite reduction required, and a fixed appliance is to be fitted, then extraction of second rather than first premolars may be more appropriate. This might save treatment time by reducing the amount of residual extraction space closure required whilst also reducing a tendency to any undesired incisor retrusion in a patient who already has a retrusive lip profile.

Treatment of the upper and lower arches is discussed separately. It is, of course, essential that treatment of the arches should be coordinated. This is discussed when the different classes of malocclusion are considered later in the text (Chapters 11–14).

The crowded lower arch

Crowded incisors and canines
Crowding is very common in this area and it tends to become worse with age, in part due to mesial drift of the buccal segments but more importantly due to the uprighting of the lower incisors that occurs during the later stages of facial

growth. If the crowding is very mild and the lower arch is not crowded elsewhere, it may be best to accept the irregularity: recent research has shown this area to be prone to long-term relapse, especially where the initial crowding was mild. However, if crowding is appreciable, extractions should be undertaken. Provided that the lower canines are mesially inclined, the extraction of lower first premolars will usually be followed by satisfactory spontaneous alignment of the labial segment. Any residual space will be taken up by forward drift of the buccal segments.

Extractions are best undertaken after the lower canines have emerged through the alveolar mucosa but before they have reached the occlusal level. However, the lower canines commonly erupt before the first premolars and so this is not always possible. Should crowding be very severe so that most or all of the extraction space is required, a space maintainer should be fitted. The degree of spontaneous space closure should be assessed approximately six months after extraction and, where necessary, an active appliance should be prescribed if full closure is a treatment aim.

Where the lower canines are distally inclined, spontaneous resolution of lower incisor crowding will not follow the extraction of first premolars, and lower fixed appliance treatment to retract the canines is usually indicated. Where a lower canine is crowded it is sometimes tempting to extract this tooth. However, the approximal contact between a lower lateral incisor and first premolar is rarely satisfactory due to the shape of the teeth and so extraction of a lower canine should be avoided if at all possible.

Although it often seems to offer a simple solution to lower incisor crowding, normally the extraction of a lower incisor should be avoided for the following reasons:

- Crowding frequently reappears amongst the remaining three incisors.
- The lower intercanine width decreases and this may lead to a secondary reduction in upper intercanine width with crowding in the upper labial segment.
- Usually it is not possible to fit four upper incisors around three lower incisors: either an increase in overjet or upper incisor crowding may have to be accepted unless the upper canines can be retracted beyond their normal relationship with the lower canines.

However, in a few well-defined cases, listed below, the extraction of a lower incisor may be appropriate, although some of the problems mentioned above still apply:

- Where one lower incisor is completely excluded from the arch and there are satisfactory approximal contacts between the other incisors.
- Where one lower incisor is damaged (e.g. fractured) or where there is extensive periodontal recession so that its long-term survival is in doubt. Fixed appliances are usually required to close the space in such circumstances.
- Where one lower incisor is severely malpositioned so that appliance treatment would present problems. Fixed appliances are still usually necessary to achieve space closure and alignment of the other teeth.
- Where the lower canines are severely distally inclined and the lower incisors are fanned there may be a case for extracting a lower incisor. However,

alignment of the remaining incisors requires fixed appliance treatment and it is usually preferable in these cases to extract first premolars and use fixed appliances to retract and upright the canines.

As may be seen from the comments above the extraction of a lower incisor is not straightforward and will most often require the addition of a fixed appliance to achieve an acceptable result. On specific occasions a lower incisor extraction may be appropriate, for example in an adult adjunctive treatment. However, it should be remembered that mild crowding of the lower incisors will usually appear better in the long term than any residual dark spaces.

In cases of mild lower incisor crowding, usually when presenting in the adult, enamel stripping, whereby the mesiodistal width of the incisors or canines is reduced, may provide just sufficient space for alignment with a local fixed appliance.

Crowded lower premolars

Where there has been early loss of deciduous molars, space loss may follow so that the premolars are crowded. It will commonly be the second premolar which is short of space since it usually erupts later than the first. The second premolar may become impacted between the first premolar and first permanent molar or be deflected lingually. If space loss is slight and the second premolar erupts before the second permanent molar, it may force its way into the arch by driving the first molar distally or by forcing the anterior teeth mesially so that incisor crowding increases. Sometimes it is appropriate to fit a lower removable appliance to move the first molar distally. This may be undertaken more readily following extraction of the lower second permanent molar (see below).

In the majority of cases, space loss is moderate and there may also be crowding of the lower incisors. In these circumstances, extraction of the first premolar may be indicated. Extraction of the second premolar does not usually allow a satisfactory spontaneous approximal contact between the first premolar and first permanent molar: the teeth tip towards one another and a stagnation area is created between them unless a fixed appliance is placed.

Where space loss has been severe so that there is already an approximal contact between the first premolar and first permanent molar, the extraction of the second premolar is advised. Severe space loss of the type mentioned above usually follows very early loss of the second deciduous molar, allowing the first permanent molar to erupt too far forwards. In these circumstances, the first permanent molar is reasonably upright and an acceptable approximal contact with the first premolar is present.

Crowded lower molars

Impaction of lower first or second permanent molars is rare and probably reflects an abnormal developmental position of the tooth rather than crowding. However, crowding of third molars is very common and, unless other permanent teeth are missing or have been extracted, there is rarely room to accommodate them in the arch. If the lower arch is otherwise regular, the extraction of the crowded third molar itself could appear to be the most suitable treatment. This could be undertaken either by a lateral approach at the time of crown completion or by conventional surgical techniques when about two-thirds of the roots have formed. However, increasingly, the limited evidence available suggests that there are few situations where asymptomatic third molars should be removed. No research has clearly demonstrated that impacted third molars are a cause of lower incisor crowding. The contemporary approach to the problem is to consider surgical removal of the third molars if they are causing symptoms or alternatively as part of a definitive treatment, perhaps for lower arch alignment.

Extraction of lower second permanent molars to provide space for crowded third molars is not usually indicated since the position of eruption of the third molar is variable and it will rarely move spontaneously into a position as good as that originally occupied by the second molar. However, where a small amount of space is also required in the second premolar region or where the second permanent molar is extensively carious, its removal may be indicated. Timing is important. For the best results (Figure 9.2), the second molar should be removed just after root formation of the third molar has started, usually between 12 and 14 years of age. It is important that the third molar is in a favourable position: it should be slightly mesially inclined, its long axis forming an angle of less than 30° to the long axis of the second molar. However, as mentioned above, even when the timing of extraction of the second molar is correct and the starting position of the third molar favourable, it is not possible to guarantee a good result.

First permanent molars are rarely the teeth of choice for orthodontic extraction. However, where one or more of these teeth are extensively carious and the long-term prognosis is questionable their removal must be considered. This is discussed in more detail in Chapters 8 and 17.

The crowded upper arch

Crowded incisors and canines
As in the case of the lower arch and provided that the canines are mesially inclined, extraction of first premolars usually gives the most satisfactory result. For maximum spontaneous improvement of crowding, the first premolars should be extracted after the canines have emerged into the mouth but before they have

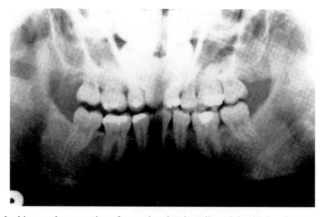

Figure 9.2 In this case the extraction of second molars has allowed the third molars to erupt into a good position

reached the occlusal level. They should not be retracted with an appliance until they have reached the occlusal level. Care should be taken to ensure that forward drift of the buccal segments does not encroach on the space required for the canines. If space is short a space maintainer should be fitted, and this is very effective in this situation.

Sometimes in crowded cases, there is a good approximal contact between the permanent upper lateral incisor and first premolar with the canine completely excluded from the arch. In these cases, extraction of the canine should be considered. The upper canine is slightly wider than the first premolar and extraction of the premolar will not provide sufficient space to accommodate the canine. If the canine is distally inclined or palatally placed and it is possible to obtain a satisfactory contact between the lateral incisor and first premolar by simple orthodontic treatment, extraction of the canine should again be considered. To improve the appearance it may be necessary to grind down the palatal cusp of the first premolar. A problem arises if the buccal surface of the first premolar is distally rotated since the appearance may then be rather poor. In these circumstances fixed appliance treatment may be required, either to align the premolar after extraction of the canine or to align the canine following extraction of the premolar. The treatment of choice depends on the features of the individual case.

If a lateral incisor is crowded into lingual occlusion with the apex palatally displaced and if the canine is erupting in a forward position and is upright or distally inclined, consideration may be given to extraction of the lateral incisor itself. The presence of a canine adjacent to a central incisor does not usually give an ideal appearance and, where possible, it is preferable to extract the first premolar or the canine to provide space for the lateral incisor. However, fixed appliance treatment would be required to move the lateral incisor apex forwards. If the patient is unsuitable for or is unwilling to wear fixed appliances, the simple expedient of extracting the lateral incisor may be justified.

Crowded upper premolars

As in the case of the lower arch, it is usually the second premolar that is crowded. If there is a good approximal contact between the first premolar and first permanent molar, the second premolar should be extracted. However, where the first premolar and first permanent molar are not in contact and particularly if there is also incisor or canine crowding, the first premolar should be removed to make space for the alignment of the second premolar. Where crowding is very mild, it may be possible to make space for the crowded second premolar by moving back the first permanent molar with an appliance, possibly following extraction of the second permanent molar (see below).

Crowded upper permanent molars

In the developing dentition, crowding of the upper molars will be manifest as 'stacking' (see Figure 9.1). When they erupt crowded molars are usually distally and buccally inclined.

Impaction of upper first permanent molars against the second deciduous molars is a result of their abnormal developmental position rather than crowding. First permanent molars are not usually the teeth of choice for orthodontic extraction. Treatment planning, where the extraction of these teeth is necessitated because of their poor life expectancy, is discussed in Chapter 8.

It is usually the third permanent molars that are crowded and if the arch is otherwise well aligned these teeth should be extracted on eruption. If more space is required to allow retraction of the upper buccal segments and provided that third molars are present, of normal size, and in favourable positions, upper second molars may be extracted. In contrast with the lower arch, the third molar will usually erupt to obtain a satisfactory contact relationship with the first permanent molar although on occasions this tooth may rotate around a large palatal root as it descends forwards along the curve of Spee.

Serial extractions

This is a procedure where, in order to encourage the spontaneous alignment of crowded incisors, the timely removal of certain deciduous and permanent teeth is undertaken. The classic approach is as follows:

1. The four deciduous canines are removed as the upper permanent lateral incisors are erupting (at about eight years of age); the alignment of the incisors should improve at the expense of space for the permanent canines.
2. The first deciduous molars are removed in order to encourage the early eruption of the first premolars. This will be most successful if the premolar roots have half formed (at about nine years of age). It is desirable that the first premolars should erupt in advance of the canines although this is often not the case in the lower arch.
3. When the lower permanent canines have just emerged through the oral mucosa, the first premolars should be extracted. This is the most important stage of the serial extraction procedure. Therefore it is important to recheck that the case is suitable for treatment by extraction of first premolars: all teeth must be present and sound; the permanent canines must be mesially inclined; and there must be crowding sufficient to justify the extraction of first premolars. If these conditions do not apply the case must be treated on its merits: the fact that serial extractions have been started by removal of deciduous canines does not commit one to going through with this line of treatment.

The full serial extraction procedure has several disadvantages:

- The child is subjected to extractions on a number of occasions and certainly multiple general anaesthetics are not justified.
- The lower permanent canine may erupt ahead of the first premolar into the extraction space of the first deciduous molar, impacting the premolar and making its removal difficult.
- Frequently, the patient requires appliance treatment anyway.

In spite of the disadvantages and limitations of 'serial extractions' as a technique, the principle of timing extractions to take advantage of spontaneous tooth movements is still valid. The removal of deciduous canines under a local anaesthetic to allow spontaneous alignment of crowded incisors may simplify later appliance treatment; and the extraction of a first premolar, before a crowded, mesially inclined canine has fully erupted, allows it to drift into the line of the arch without appliance treatment. However, the practice of extracting first deciduous molars in order to encourage the eruption of the first premolars should be carefully considered: in certain circumstances it might be valid; however, such extractions are often performed to little purpose.

Further reading

Bishara, S.E., Khadivai, P. and Kakobsen, J.R. (1995). Changes in tooth size–arch length relation-ships from the deciduous to the permanent dentition: a longitudinal study. *American Journal of Orthodontics and Dentofacial Orthopedics*, **108**, 607–13.

Proffit, W.R. (1986). On the aetiology of malocclusion. *British Journal of Orthodontics*, **13**, 1–11.

Proffit, W.R. (2000). The aetiology of orthodontic problems. In *Contemporary Orthodontics*, Chapter 5. St Louis: C.V. Mosby.

Chapter 10

Arch malrelationships

Arch malrelationships may occur in any plane. Antero-posterior arch malrelationships form the basis of Angle's classification as described earlier in Chapter 7.

Antero-posterior malrelationships

Buccal segments

Antero-posterior malrelationships of the buccal segments often reflect antero-posterior jaw malrelationships. However, since the position of the teeth in relation to the skeletal base can vary, it is possible to find cases with normal skeletal relationships and arch malrelationships, and vice versa. When the lower buccal segment is posteriorly positioned relative to the upper, this may be referred to as a Class II buccal segment relationship or as a disto-occlusion. Where the lower buccal segment is forward in relation to the upper, this is a Class III buccal segment relationship or mesio-occlusion.

Labial segments

The labial segment relationship often, but not always, follows the buccal segment relationship. For example, it is possible to find a case with a Class II incisor relationship but a Class I or even Class III buccal segment relationship.

The aetiology and treatment of the different antero-posterior arch malrelationships are discussed in Chapters 11–14.

Vertical malrelationships

Buccal segments

Vertical malrelationships are not common in the buccal segments. Where the intermaxillary height is increased and there is a skeletal anterior open bite (Figure 10.1) this may extend into the buccal segments so that perhaps only the most posterior molar teeth are in occlusion. In these cases there is a lateral open bite as well as an anterior open bite. Occasionally a lateral open bite is found in isolation from any other occlusal anomaly. The reasons for this are usually obscure but there may be a localized failure of alveolar development.

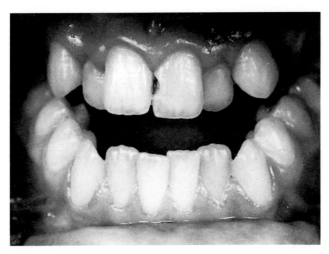

Figure 10.1 This patient has a Class III malocclusion with a skeletal anterior open bite and a bilateral crossbite. These occlusal malrelationships reflect skeletal malrelationships: there is a Class III skeletal pattern; the lower facial third is increased in height; and the maxilla is narrow relative to the mandible

Over-eruption of buccal teeth that are unopposed or occlude against a submerging deciduous tooth are, of course, seen quite commonly.

Labial segments

In normal occlusion the lower incisors occlude with the cingulum plateau of the upper incisors and the overbite is one-third to one-half of the height of the lower incisor crowns.

Increase in overbite
Skeletal factors. It is often stated that a small lower facial height is associated with a deep overbite. However, this is not a constant relationship and occlusal factors (see below) must also play a part.

Occlusal factors. Where there is no incisor contact due to a large overjet (Class II Division 1), the lower incisors will often erupt until they contact the palatal mucosa and the overbite will be deep. Where there is an adaptive anterior oral seal between tongue and lower lip, the overbite is incomplete but is still deep in most cases (see Chapter 5).

Where the overjet is normal and the incisors are retroclined (Class II Division 2), so that the interincisor angle is increased, the overbite will also be increased. This may happen developmentally or as a result of an inappropriate treatment of a severe Class II Division 1 incisor relationship with removable appliances so that the upper incisors are over-retroclined. Even if the overbite has been reduced during treatment, it will increase again when appliances are discarded.

The reduction of a deep overbite will be stable only if at the end of treatment the lower incisors occlude with the palatal surfaces of the upper incisors, the interincisor angle is within the normal range, and the teeth are in a position of labiolingual balance.

Reduction in overbite

If there is a mild Class III incisor relationship with occlusal contact between the upper and lower incisors, the overbite will be reduced.

An overbite may be reduced and incomplete for a variety of reasons, which are dealt with in the following section.

Anterior open bite

Here there is no occlusal contact between the incisors, and the upper incisors do not overlap the lowers in the vertical plane. Anterior open bite is discussed below according to its aetiology: skeletal, soft tissue, habit and miscellaneous.

Skeletal factors. Where the anterior intermaxillary space is increased, the vertical growth of the labial segments may be insufficient to achieve tooth contact when the posterior teeth are brought into occlusion (Figure 10.1). In the most severe cases only the last standing teeth will meet in occlusion. Generally, the Frankfort–mandibular planes angle is increased and frequently, but not always, there is a Class III skeletal pattern.

It is interesting that except in the most severe cases, the open bite is seldom of concern to the patient either aesthetically or functionally. Frequently, of course, coexisting features such as mandibular protrusion do worry the patient. Correction of the anterior open bite by orthodontic means alone is rarely indicated. Appliance therapy to elongate the incisors will rarely be successful. Extraction or grinding of posterior teeth is definitely contraindicated since the patient will then be forced to overclose into occlusion, exaggerating any prominence of the mandible and possibly giving rise to muscle pain at a later date. Overlay dentures are contraindicated because of the problems of food stagnation and because they rarely improve the appearance of this type of patient. The only successful treatment is surgery (see Chapter 22), although such an approach is valid only in highly motivated patients. Of course, if surgery to correct a Class III skeletal pattern is to be undertaken it should be planned to deal with the open bite at the same time.

Soft tissue factors. Where there is an anterior open bite due to other aetiological factors (e.g. a habit) the tongue will frequently come forwards to fill the gap. This is purely an adaptive pattern of behaviour. A tongue-to-lip anterior oral seal (see Chapter 5) is usually associated with an incomplete overbite. The tongue behaviour will re-adapt on correction of the overbite. In the very rare cases of a primary atypical tongue thrust, the soft tissue activity is responsible for an incomplete overbite or even an anterior open bite. As discussed in Chapter 5, these cases are difficult to diagnose and may not be suitable for orthodontic treatment.

Habits. Digit or dummy sucking may produce an anterior open bite, which will often improve spontaneously on cessation of the habit (also see Chapter 8).

Miscellaneous. The various developmental (e.g. cleft palate), pathological (e.g. bony dysplasia) and traumatic (e.g. bilateral condylar fracture) causes of anterior open bite will not be discussed here.

Transverse malrelationships

Buccal segments

A transverse malrelationship of the buccal segments is termed a 'crossbite' and this may be bilateral (Figure 10.1) or unilateral (Figure 10.2). In most cases of crossbite the upper arch is narrow, relative to the lower, so the buccal cusps of the lower teeth overlap the buccal cusps of the uppers. Occasionally, a lingual crossbite or 'scissors bite' is found in which the upper teeth completely overlap the lowers buccally.

Bilateral crossbite

This is a symmetrical transverse arch malrelationship and is usually skeletal in origin. The maxilla is narrow in relation to the mandible and this is reflected in the arch widths. Bilateral crossbites are frequently found in association with severe Class III malocclusions (Figure 10.1), in part because the maxilla is often narrow relative to the mandible and in part because a broader part of the lower arch opposes a narrower part of the upper arch (due to the horizontal discrepancy).

Although from a theoretical viewpoint masticatory efficiency is reduced, in practice a bilateral crossbite is seldom of functional significance. Additionally, expansion of the upper arch to correct the crossbite is rarely stable. Thus these malocclusions are usually best left untreated. Occasionally, rapid expansion of the mid-palatal suture may be attempted using a fixed appliance. This should be undertaken only as part of a more general treatment plan, and although expansion of the suture may be stable, occlusal relapse may still follow.

Unilateral crossbite

It is important to distinguish between unilateral crossbites with lateral displacement and those without.

With displacement (Figure 10.2). In most non-pathological cases of unilateral crossbite, when the mandible is at rest, the arches are symmetrical. However,

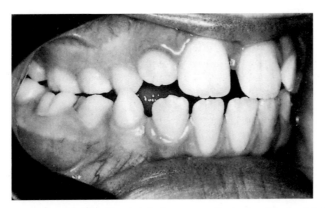

Figure 10.2 A unilateral crossbite. Note that the lower centre line is also off to the right. In centric relation this patient's buccal teeth would meet cusp to cusp, and so there is a lateral displacement to the right in order to obtain maximal occlusion

both arches have the same relative width and with normal hinge closure the cheek teeth would meet cusp to cusp. In order to achieve maximal intercuspation, the mandible is displaced to one side so that there is an apparently asymmetrical malocclusion. Generally, the midlines of the arches will be coincident at rest (before contact), but in occlusion the lower midline will be displaced to the side of the crossbite.

The aetiology of this type of occlusion may be a transverse skeletal discrepancy, similar to but less severe than the type causing a bilateral crossbite (i.e. the maxilla may be narrow relative to the mandible and there may be a mild Class III skeletal pattern). However, a unilateral crossbite of this type may be caused by soft tissue factors. For example, if swallowing habitually takes place without occlusion of the teeth, pressure from the cheeks may equalize the widths of the arches. Similarly, with habits such as persistent digit sucking, forces from the cheeks whilst the teeth are not in occlusion may narrow the maxillary arch so that a unilateral crossbite with mandibular displacement occurs.

The amount of expansion of the upper arch necessary to correct the crossbite is small and, unlike a bilateral crossbite, the occlusion of the teeth will normally prevent relapse. As the maxillary arch is basically symmetrical the expansion should be bilateral.

Without displacement. Here there is a true asymmetry of one arch which will often reflect an underlying skeletal asymmetry. This may be within normal limits but occasionally it is produced by some pathological factor. For example, unilateral cleft palate produces a maxillary asymmetry, whilst unilateral condylar hyperplasia may produce a mandibular asymmetry with secondary occlusal effects.

Clearly, where the crossbite is produced by some pathological factor, treatment considerations will primarily be directed towards the basic anomaly although occlusal factors are also important (cleft palate is discussed in Chapter 23).

A unilateral crossbite without displacement in an individual with an otherwise normal occlusion does not usually require treatment but, if treatment is undertaken, it may be unstable.

Chapter 11

Class I malocclusions

Class I malocclusions are by far the most common problem, accounting for about half of all malocclusions.

Occlusal and dento-alveolar features

Labial segments

In a Class I incisor relationship, the lower incisor edges should occlude with or lie directly below the cingulum plateau of the upper incisors (Figure 11.1). This relationship need not apply to all the incisors: for example, there may be local irregularities such as rotations or there may be one or two instanding upper incisors. However, taking the labial segments as a whole, there should be a normal antero-posterior relationship between them.

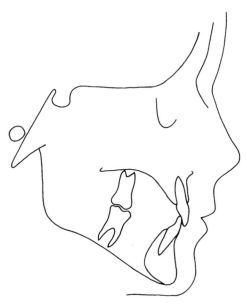

Figure 11.1 A Class I malocclusion associated with a Class I skeletal pattern

Buccal segments

There may be any type of molar relationship present. This will depend on the teeth that have been lost previously. The buccal segments may be asymmetrical due to earlier asymmetrical tooth loss. This, in turn, may produce a centre-line shift. Because of the order of eruption, if there is a crowded dental arch, the last tooth within the arch to erupt will often be impacted or crowded out of the line of the dental arch. Mandibular second premolars often have a vertical impaction, and maxillary canines are frequently buccally excluded.

Skeletal relationships

Antero-posterior

The skeletal pattern is usually Class I (Figure 11.1), but it is possible to find a Class I malocclusion in association with a Class II or Class III skeletal pattern provided that the inclinations of the teeth, and their positions on the skeletal bases, compensate for the skeletal malrelationship.

Vertical and transverse

The jaw relationships in the vertical and transverse planes are usually within the normal range but there may be malrelationships in these planes and associated occlusal anomalies.

Mandibular positions and paths of closure

Displacement of a single tooth from arch line due to crowding may give rise to a premature contact with the opposing arch and lead to a displacement on closure. (See also Chapters 8 and 10.)

Soft tissues

As in the case of the skeletal relationships, the soft tissue form and activity are usually within the normal range.

Growth

For Class I malocclusion there will be harmonious growth between the maxilla and mandible which maintains the skeletal relationships in all three planes.

Oral health

As with most malocclusions, except in specific circumstances, a Class I malocclusion, *per se*, does not pose a specific threat to the long-term dental health of the individual. There are one or two exceptions:

1. *Incisor crossbite*. A lingually placed upper incisor may suffer abrasion on its labial surface from its opposing tooth which, in turn, may be displaced labially with loss of periodontal support.
2. *Localized problems*. Partially erupted or impacted teeth, or severely imbricated teeth, may create local stagnation areas where plaque removal is particularly difficult, even for the oral hygiene enthusiast! This can lead to the two major plaque-related diseases of caries and periodontal disease.

Treatment aims

The aims of treatment can be summarized as follows:

1. To improve the aesthetics of the teeth and the function of the teeth and jaws.
2. To relieve crowding and produce alignment of the teeth within the arches.
3. If necessary, to reduce a deepened overbite and improve the interincisal angle.

Treatment planning

Treatment of the upper and lower arches must be coordinated. The general aims of treatment will be relief of crowding and alignment of the teeth. As a rule, it is simplest to plan treatment of the lower arch first, then to build the upper arch around the lower. Usually the size and form of the lower arch must be accepted if the result is to be stable. As a general rule in Class I cases, if extractions are necessary in the lower arch, matching teeth should be extracted from the upper arch. However, if there is an asymmetrical problem (e.g. a centre-line shift), then an asymmetrical extraction pattern may be required. Usually the absence of any teeth will necessitate modifications to the treatment plan.

Treatment options

No treatment

The presence of a malocclusion does not automatically indicate a need for remedial treatment. Many mild malocclusions can and should be accepted as part of the rich variety of life. Some patients feel that mild tooth displacements lend 'character' to their smile and do not wish treatment.

Extractions

Where teeth are favourably inclined, for example mesially-tipped canines, loss of first premolars will create space for the spontaneous uprighting of the canines. Similarly, loss of lower first premolars will relieve the vertical impaction of second premolars and they should then erupt into occlusion. There can be no guarantee that this spontaneous change will occur, and the patient should be reviewed regularly.

Approximately nine months after the extractions most of the spontaneous change will have taken place and a decision will need to be taken regarding further active treatment.

Removable appliances

An upper removable appliance can tip teeth mesiodistally or labiopalatally. Provided that the initial position of the tooth is favourable for tipping, a

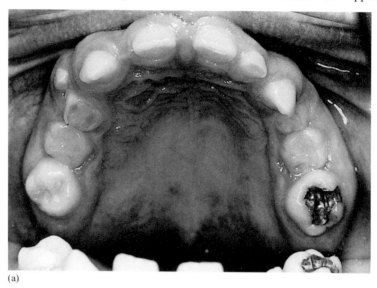

(a)

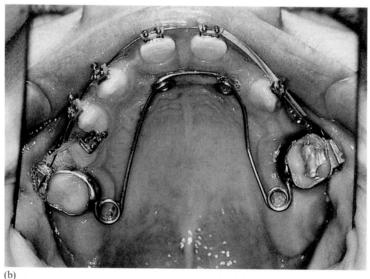

(b)

Figure 11.2 (a) Occlusal view of upper arch of patient with hypodontia. Note that both first permanent molars are rotated mesiopalatally. (b) A quad helix appliance has been attached to stainless-steel bands on the molars to derotate them, and is now being used to help stabilize these teeth whilst other work is carried out using a bonded upper fixed appliance

satisfactory result may be expected. Lower removable appliances are seldom used, as they are difficult to fit, constrict the tongue space and have limited space for the active components. Should tooth movement in the lower arch be necessary, a lower fixed appliance should be used.

Single arch fixed appliances

A common approach in the UK is the '2 × 4' single arch fixed, i.e. bands on the molars (the '2') and bonded brackets on the incisors (the '4'). This produces alignment of the anterior teeth and may be placed on the upper or lower arches. This is particularly useful if there are incisor rotations. A full single arch fixed will clearly give better control of all the teeth.

Upper and lower arch fixed appliances

There is no doubt that these give the best control of all the teeth and hence a high likelihood of a good quality result. In the severely crowded mouth with anterior and/or posterior rotations, this is the treatment of choice. Adjuncts such as a quad helix may be used to derotate molars (Figure 11.2b), or correct simple crossbites, as well as contributing to molar anchorage. Vertical control of teeth is also possible, elastics being attached to the upper and lower teeth to close down an open bite arising from a dento-alveolar problem such as a prolonged digit-sucking habit.

Functional appliances

These are rarely of assistance in the management of true Class I cases.

Orthognathic surgery

This approach is only of assistance in unusual and specific conditions, most often related to severe vertical discrepancy.

Post-treatment stability

Correction of rotations is one of the major problems of post-treatment stability. Various methods have been tried to enhance stability. (See also Chapter 25.)

Over-correction. By anticipating the relapse, over-correction of the rotated tooth should allow the tooth to settle in its correct position. It is very difficult to estimate how much over-correction will be necessary.

Pericision. This is severing of the supracrestal periodontal fibres that run between the tooth and the gingivae (see Chapter 20 and Figure 15.2). These fibres are slow to remodel (not being attached to bone), and by cutting through them the tension within the area is released, and new attachments are made with the tooth in its corrected position. This technique has failed to fulfil all its theoretical promise, although the amount of relapse is reduced in teeth which have had pericision.

Positive retention. Using a palatally or lingually bonded retainer, attached to the derotated tooth and its adjacent teeth, there should be little opportunity for rotational relapse to occur.

Long retention. Reitan showed that tension in the periodontal ligament following tooth rotation lasted for about nine months. This means that full-time retention should last for at least that long. This may be achieved in part by correcting rotations early in treatment.

Combined treatment. Any of the above in combination.

Further reading

Ahreus, D.G., Shapiro, Y. and Kuffinec, M.M. (1981). An approach to rotational relapse. *American Journal of Orthodontics*, **80**, 83–91.
Houston, W.J.B. (1989). Incisor centroid relationships and overbite depth. *European Journal of Orthodontics*, **11**, 139–43.

Chapter 12

Class II Division 1 malocclusions

After Class I malocclusions, Class II Division 1 are the most common malocclusions, accounting for between 25 and 33% of all malocclusions in a typical Western population.

Occlusal and dento-alveolar features

Labial segments

The lower incisor edges lie posterior to the cingulum plateau of the upper incisors and there is an increased overjet. The overjet may be increased due to:

- Proclined upper incisors as a result of digit-sucking, lower lip activity or developmental position.
- Retroclined lower incisors as a result of digit-sucking, lower lip activity or, in severe cases with increased overbite, the lower incisors being trapped behind the vertical part of the anterior palate.
- Skeletal Class II relationship. With a skeletal Class II relationship the lower incisors may well be proclined beyond their normal angulation, as a result of a natural attempt to compensate for the antero-posterior skeletal discrepancy. In the upper arch the incisors may be at a normal angulation to the maxillary plane.
- Any combination of the above.

The overbite is variable and may be influenced by the underlying skeletal pattern or various soft tissue factors such as tongue thrust or digit-sucking. Most commonly, the overbite is increased and complete.

Buccal segments

It is possible to have Class I buccal segments, in which case the upper incisors will be proclined or lowers retroclined. More usually the molars are Class II, with the mesiobuccal cusp of the upper first molar anterior to the mid-buccal groove of the lower first molar.

Skeletal relationships

Antero-posterior

There is usually a Class II skeletal pattern (Figure 12.1). In many cases this is the primary aetiological factor responsible for the Class II arch relationship. The more severe the skeletal malrelationship, the more severe the malocclusion is likely to be and the poorer the prognosis for orthodontic correction alone.

In a number of cases the skeletal pattern is Class I (or rarely mild Class III). In these cases, it is the position of the teeth on the skeletal bases that is at fault, due either to their developmental positions or to their inclination under the influence of the soft tissues or digit-sucking habit.

Vertical

The anterior skeletal face height is usually average, although it may be either high or more rarely low. A high angle or dolichofacial pattern is usually associated with an unfavourable facial profile with little chin prominence. Orthodontic treatment for these patients is difficult. The incisor overbite will often reflect the vertical skeletal arrangement.

Transverse

There are no characteristic transverse malrelationships.

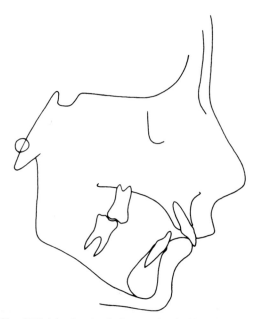

Figure 12.1 A Class II Division 1 malocclusion associated with a Class II skeletal pattern

Mandibular positions and paths of closure

In many cases the mandible is habitually in the rest position and there is a centric path of closure. In a few cases the mandible is habitually postured forwards to facilitate the production of a lip seal, the so-called 'Sunday face'. If there is a well-established postural habit, the patient will be able to close easily into their forward position, and the unwary practitioner may attempt to correct what, at first sight, appears to be a relatively mild problem. Once treatment has started, the mandibular posture will be revealed and this may present considerable treatment difficulties, especially if inappropriate teeth have been extracted. True distal displacements are rare.

Soft tissues and habits

The lips are frequently incompetent (see Figure 5.1c). This often contributes to the lack of control and consequent proclination of the upper incisors. In some cases, a lip seal will be maintained, but frequently there is a tongue-to-lower-lip seal with the lower lip lying behind the upper incisors (Figures 12.2a and 5.2). If, after retraction of the upper incisors, a lip seal will be obtained with the lower lip covering the incisal third of the upper incisor (Figure 12.2b), the outlook for stability is good. If, however, the lower lip does not control the corrected upper incisor position but a tongue-to-lower-lip anterior oral seal continues, the prognosis for treatment stability is poor.

In a very few patients there is a primary atypical swallowing behaviour (see Chapter 5). This will be an aetiological factor in producing the incisor malrelationship and will preclude a stable reduction of the overjet. In these cases the overjet should be accepted.

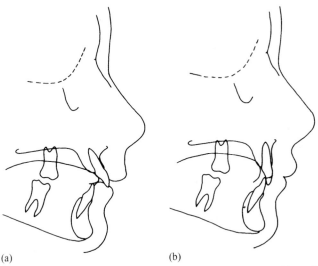

(a)   (b)

Figure 12.2 (a) An adaptive anterior oral seal with contact between tongue and lower lip. (b) Following retraction of the upper incisors, an anterior seal will be obtained by lip contact. The lower lip covers the incisal third of the upper incisors and this will ensure stability of the overjet reduction

Those patients with a reduced face height (brachyfacial) will have an everted lower lip resting on the palatal of the upper incisors, and will frequently have a strong mentalis muscle activity maintaining an oral seal (see Figure 5.1d). These can be difficult to treat as the lower lip resists the lingual movement of the upper incisors (see Figure 5.2).

There is often a history of digit-sucking and in some cases this may have contributed to the incisor malrelationship (see Chapter 8).

Growth

The differential growth rate of the two jaws is generally helpful in Class II Division 1 cases, as mandibular growth will tend to reduce the severity of the problem. Those patients with dolichofacial patterns (see Figure 5.1b) will have less favourable growth direction than the brachyfacial pattern, the former exhibiting vertical mandibular growth, the latter horizontal mandibular growth.

Oral health

An overjet in excess of 6 mm, in conjunction with incompetent lips in a 7–14-year-old boy, signifies a high risk of accidental fracture of the upper incisors. Unfortunately, unless a functional appliance is prescribed (see below and also Chapter 18), the age range during which there is the greatest risk of trauma is not normally associated with orthodontic treatment.

Incompetent lips are also often associated with hyperplastic gingivitis around the upper incisors. This is sometimes incorrectly called 'mouth-breathing gingivitis', although in fact these patients are not usually mouth-breathers (there is often an anterior oral seal between tongue and lower lip and a posterior seal between the soft palate and dorsum of the tongue). The gingivitis is a result of the drying out of the oral mucosa due to the lack of lip cover.

Although in some cases with a deep, complete overbite the lower incisors occlude directly with the palatal mucosa, trauma is surprisingly rare.

Treatment aims

The aims of treatment can be summarized as follows:

1. To improve the aesthetics of the teeth and the function of the teeth and jaws.
2. To relieve crowding and produce alignment of the teeth within the dental arches.
3. To reduce the overjet but not at the expense of worsening the upper lip contour. (Beware over-retracting the upper incisors to match a true mandibular arch retrusion.)
4. To reduce the overbite and achieve a stable interincisal angle, if necessary applying palatal root torque to the upper incisors.
5. To achieve a good intercuspation between upper and lower buccal teeth. This would usually be Class I, but could be Class II (see below).

Treatment planning

The primary objectives of treatment are to relieve crowding and to correct the incisor relationship. Attention should also be paid to the buccal segment relationship. In the interests of stability and occlusal function, there should be a good intercuspation between the upper and lower teeth. A Class II buccal segment relationship (which may result if premolar extractions are undertaken only in the upper arch) is, on occasions, acceptable provided that the intercuspation is good. It is a prerequisite of any orthodontic treatment plan that the number, location and long-term prognosis of all teeth are confirmed, most particularly if tooth extraction is envisaged.

The lower arch

The lower arch should be planned first. Under most circumstances the antero-posterior position of the lower incisors, and the intercanine width must be accepted. Proclination of lower incisors is only acceptable if they are clearly held in a retroclined position. This means that if there is crowding, teeth usually will have to be extracted. Research has shown that the lower intercanine width is stable after the age of about nine years, and alteration of this dimension will not be stable. Space will also be required in the lower arch in order to level the curve of Spee, which is frequently increased when the overbite is deep. Without extractions, space for lower arch levelling can only come from such spacing as may already be present, or arch expansion such as lower incisor proclination or molar retroclination. Transverse expansion is rarely indicated.

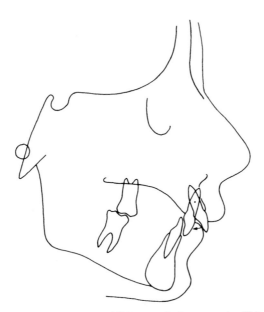

Figure 12.3 When the overjet is large and if the upper incisors are not sufficiently proclined, retraction with a removable appliance will produce a Class II Division 2 incisor relationship

The upper arch

The upper anterior teeth are much more amenable to permanent and stable alteration of their positions. Thus, the upper arch should be built around the lower arch. If lower extractions are required, then upper extractions will be necessary. Particular attention should be paid to the post-treatment incisor inclination; where tipping of the incisor leads to a retroclined final position, bodily movement and/or torque with a fixed appliance should be planned for, and the necessary anchorage requirements considered in the initial plan. A Class II Division 1 incisor relationship should never be converted to a Class II Division 2 pattern by treatment (Figure 12.3).

Treatment options

No treatment

A mild Class II Division 1 incisor relationship may be considered quite attractive, and correction of the problem should only be considered if there are clear oral health or psychological reasons.

Extractions only

This is rarely successful. Loss of teeth will relieve crowding, but has no benefit to the antero-posterior incisor relationship. In fact, if anything, loss of lower premolars will encourage some mild retroclination of lower incisors, which would increase the overjet. In the lower arch, if extractions are necessary, increased mesial crown tip of the canines must be present so that these teeth may upright spontaneously into the extraction site. Residual space should close by mesial movement of the posterior teeth. On occasions, as a compromise, totally buccally excluded teeth may be extracted when no other treatment is planned.

Removable appliances

If the upper incisors are proclined, and the maxillary canines have an increased mesiodistal tip, then removable appliance mechanics can produce a satisfactory result. Remember that if lower canines will be moving distally, the amount of distal movement necessary for the upper canines to achieve a Class I relationship will be increased, and this may influence the choice of treatment mechanics.

Typically, treatment of Class II Division 1 using removable appliances will involve the following stages:

1. Extraction of first premolars: $\frac{4/4}{4/4}$.
2. Upper removable appliance with:

    - Adams clasps on the first molars
    - Southend clasp on the incisors

- canine retraction springs (these may be buccally or palatally approaching, depending on the labiopalatal position of the canine)
- an anterior biting platform for overbite reduction.

Once the canines have been moved distally into a Class I relationship with the lower canines, a second appliance for overjet reduction and maintenance of overbite reduction will be needed as follows:

- Adams clasps on molars
- soft wire spurs to mesial of $\underline{3/3}$
- wire spring (e.g. Roberts retractor) to reduce overjet (for a full range of labial bows suitable for palatal tipping of upper incisors see Adams and Kerr, 1990)
- anterior biting platform to maintain overbite reduction.

The acrylic should be trimmed progressively from behind the upper incisors to provide space for their palatal movement. In trimming the bite plane to allow upper incisor retraction (see Figure 16.11), it is important to clear it well away from these teeth yet to maintain contact with the lower incisors and provide space for the palatal mucosa to move back. This is because the soft tissues remodel at a much slower rate than the hard tissues. The wire spurs to the canines will have to be removed in the later stages of treatment to allow contact between canine and lateral incisor.

Once overjet reduction is complete the same appliance with a passive labial bow may be used as a retainer. Alternatively, a third retainer appliance will be necessary:

- Adams clasps on first molars
- Hawley bow.

This should be worn full time for 4–6 months followed by a period of nocturnal retention. (See also Chapter 16 for further details on appliance construction and use.)

Anchorage control
There is no such thing as a static anchor point, unless an implant or ankylosed tooth is used. It is important therefore to be able to assess the amount of anchorage loss that is occurring. There are a variety of ways in which anchorage loss (i.e. in these circumstances unwanted mesial movement of the upper molars) may be judged:

Reduction in canine–molar distance. Progress of distal movement of canines is often recorded by measuring from a reproducible point on the canine, such as the cusp tip, back to another reproducible point on the molar, such as the mid-buccal groove. During treatment this distance should reduce and this may be brought about by:

- distal movement of the canine (desirable), or
- mesial movement of the molar, which is undesirable anchorage loss.

Canine relationship. If the canine is moving distally, and provided that there have been no lower arch extractions, there will be a change in the canine relationship towards Class I. However, if there have been lower arch extractions the lower canines will also be moving distally spontaneously, consequently there may be little or no change in canine relationship for some time and this may mask loss of anchorage control.

Molar relationship. If no lower arch extractions have been carried out, mesial movement of the upper molar will result in a change in the molar relationship. However, if lower extractions were carried out, then mesial movement of the upper molar may go undetected, as the lower molar will also move mesially.

Overjet. If the molars move mesially during canine retraction, the baseplate of the appliance, which is attached to the molars via the Adams clasps, will also move mesially. Contact of the baseplate with the palatal of the upper incisors will, in turn, mean that these teeth will be pushed forwards with a consequent increase in overjet. This is probably the most reliable means of monitoring anchorage loss. It must be remembered, however, that the presence of an anterior biting platform will rotate the mandible downwards and slightly backwards, and this in itself will produce a small increase in the overjet. The overjet should always be measured with the appliance out of the mouth, and with the mandible in maximum retrusion.

For methods of anchorage reinforcement and control see Chapter 16.

Bimaxillary proclination

Correction of a Class II Division 1 malocclusion in which there is an increased and complete overbite and proclined lower incisors, as in a significant bimaxillary proclination, should not be attempted using removable appliances. The resolution of forces on the lower incisors from the anterior biting platform will tend to procline these teeth even further, and prevent full overbite reduction (Figure 12.4). This is an unstable situation and will lead to failure of treatment.

Single arch fixed appliance

The use of a single arch fixed appliance to correct a Class II Division 1 malocclusion can only be attempted where there is no overbite problem, and is indicated where the angulations of the canines are unfavourable for tooth tipping

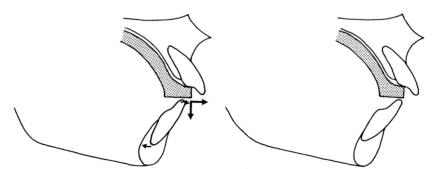

Figure 12.4 The unwanted effects of an anterior biting platform on a removable appliance used in a bimaxillary proclination case. The effect of the biting platform on the lower incisor is to produce a small amount of intrusion, and some further proclination of the tooth. This will be self-limiting when the root meets the lingual cortical plate of bone. The overall effect is an unexpected reduction in overjet caused by lower incisor proclination, which is unstable and liable to relapse when the appliance is withdrawn

and/or there are incisor rotations. The need for headgear is also increased, as intermaxillary anchorage reinforcement is impossible in the absence of a lower appliance.

Upper and lower arch fixed appliances

This treatment has the ability to deliver the highest quality of result in the majority of cases. Control of all the teeth in all planes of space is possible, and the opportunity to use intermaxillary traction to reinforce anchorage can often obviate the need for headgear. Use of fixed appliances is indicated where any of the following conditions exist:

• the angulation of the canines is unsuitable for simple tipping
• the upper incisors are already at their correct inclination to the maxillary plane
• there are anterior and/or posterior rotations
• the lower incisors are proclined or retroclined
• the malocclusion is more severe
• controlled space closure of residual space in the extraction site is required
• there is an increased and complete overbite in an adult
• multiple and/or three-dimensional tooth movements are necessary.

Functional appliances

Use of a functional appliance is appropriate in specific circumstances:

• there must be two well-aligned arches
• there must be average face height/maxillary : mandibular planes angle
• there should be some proclination of the upper incisors, and minimal proclination of the lower incisors
• there should be a noticeable improvement in the facial profile when the patient postures the mandible forwards
• the patient should not yet have entered their adolescent growth spurt
• it must be accepted that further treatment using other forms of mechanics may be necessary.

See Chapter 18 for a full discussion of functional appliances.

Orthognathic surgery

Severe skeletal discrepancies will not allow the usual dento-alveolar camouflage that orthodontic treatment can produce. A combined orthodontic/orthognathic surgical approach is required. This essentially involves alignment of each arch individually to produce correct tooth relationships and inclinations within each arch. The arch relationships are then surgically corrected and some further orthodontic treatment will be required to settle the teeth into a suitable final occlusal arrangement. This requires careful planning by both the orthodontist and the maxillofacial surgeon for a successful outcome. See Chapter 22 for further details.

Post-treatment stability

The aim of treatment is to bring the upper incisors under control of the lower lip. This usually means that the lower lip should overlap the incisal third of the upper incisor. If this lip control cannot be achieved, some form of permanent retention may be necessary. This may take the form of a Hawley retainer worn on alternate nights, or a bonded palatal retainer attached to the six upper anterior teeth.

Further reading

Adams, C.P. and Kerr, W.J.S. (1990). *The Design and Use of Removable Appliances*, 6th edn. Oxford: Butterworth-Heinemann.

Houston, W.J.B. and Walters, N.R.E. (1977). The design of buccal canine retraction springs for removable orthodontic appliances. *British Journal of Orthodontics*, **4**, 191–5.

Muir, J.D. and Reed, R.T. (1979). *Tooth Movements with Removable Appliances*. London: Pitman Medical.

Chapter 13

Class II Division 2 malocclusions

Class II Division 2 malocclusions occur in approximately 7 to 10% of a Western (largely Caucasian-based) population.

Occlusal and dento-alveolar features

According to Angle's classification, in a Class II Division 2 malocclusion the lower arch should be at least one-half cusp width postnormal to the upper, and the upper central incisors should be retroclined (see Figure 7.3). The upper lateral incisors may be similarly retroclined although in other cases, particularly in the presence of crowding, they may be proclined.

Labial segments

The amount of retroclination of the upper central incisors is closely related to the degree of postnormality of the lower arch, which is, in turn, related to the severity of the skeletal malrelationship. The upper lateral incisors, when proclined, are typically mesially inclined and mesiolabially rotated (see Figure 7.3). Otherwise they may be retroclined in a line with the central incisors.

The lower labial segment is frequently retroclined, in sympathy with the uppers, a feature that may contribute to lower incisor crowding but also increases the interincisor angle and so has an adverse effect on the depth of overbite. Often the overbite is worsened by a tendency to dento-alveolar vertical excess of both upper and lower labial segments. In such a presentation typically the lower curve of Spee is increased, whilst in the upper jaw the patient may appear to have a 'gummy smile'.

The overjet is usually only slightly increased, the distal position of the lower arch being compensated for by the retroclination of the upper central incisors. In severe cases, where there is a marked Class II skeletal pattern, the overjet may be larger. In this type of case the overbite tends to be deep and complete, the depth of overbite depending on the severity of the skeletal malrelationship and the size of the interincisor angle.

In the majority of patients presenting with this malocclusion the overbite is only mildly or moderately increased but on occasions it can be very deep, with the lower incisors occluding on the palatal mucosa and the upper incisors on the gingivae labial to the lower incisors. In the presence of poor oral hygiene there can be severe soft tissue inflammation associated with such a presentation. Fortunately – for they are quite difficult to treat – these severe cases are quite rare. Most Class II Division 2 cases are mild with a deep, but not excessive, overbite.

Buccal segments

These may be crowded if there has been early loss of deciduous molar teeth with forward drift of the first permanent molars. Lateral or vertical exclusion from the dental arch of the second permanent premolars is not uncommon.

Skeletal relationships

Antero-posterior

The skeletal pattern is usually Class I or mild Class II (Figure 13.1). The profile is frequently well balanced, although tending to a bimaxillary retroclination, with the chin in a good relationship with the rest of the face.

The receding chin, so often seen in Class II Division 1 cases, is not common in Class II Division 2. These malocclusions are not usually associated with severe Class II skeletal patterns unless the malocclusion is a result of an inappropriate treatment where the upper incisors in a severe Class II Division 1 case have been tipped back to reduce the overjet (see Figure 12.3). In the patient presenting with a true Class II Division 2 with a significant skeletal discrepancy, studies employing lateral cephalograms have found the cause of the discrepancy often to be an increase in the length of the anterior cranial base. This leads to a more distal positioning of the glenoid fossa and thus the mandible.

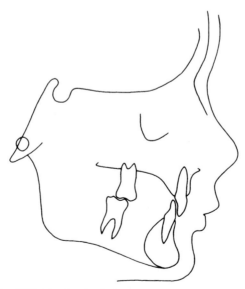

Figure 13.1 A Class II Division 2 malocclusion associated with a mild Class II skeletal pattern

Vertical

The lower facial height is reduced or average. The Frankfort–mandibular planes angle is often low, this reading frequently being accentuated by an upward canting of the distal part of the maxillary plane. The low anterior facial height may contribute to the depth of overbite.

Transverse

There are no characteristic malrelationships. However, in rarer presentations with a large skeletal discrepancy, a 'scissors bite' (with upper buccal teeth occluding outside lowers) may be present.

Mandibular positions and paths of closure

In many cases, the habitual position of the mandible is the rest position and the path of closure into occlusion is a simple hinge movement. In some of the more severe cases, however, the mandible is habitually postured downwards and forwards. The reasons for this are obscure but it is important to recognize that the upward and backward path of closure in these cases is a deviation into a position of centric occlusion and is not a distal displacement. True posterior displacements are sometimes found in Class II Division 2 cases, particularly where there has been loss of posterior teeth. These patients will often present with pain in early adult life. Attrition facets will be observed on certain teeth. Careful occlusal analysis and equilibration are necessary.

Soft tissues

The lips are held together, usually with minimal circumoral contraction. The lip line is often high, the lower lip covering more than the occlusal half of the upper incisors, a factor which is often important in the aetiology of the condition (see Chapter 5). In some cases there may be an accentuated labiomental fold, and an increased nasio-labial angle, with flattening of the upper lip profile is a frequent finding.

Variations in swallowing behaviour are not usually important in the aetiology or treatment of this malocclusion.

Growth

Many patients with this type of malocclusion exhibit a closing growth rotation (see Chapter 3). This will contribute to the reduced facial height and the deep overbite tendency. It may also make the reduction of the overbite more difficult during treatment necessitating true intrusion of the lower incisors, by means of a fixed appliance to reduce (flatten) the curve of Spee.

Tooth morphology

A common finding in this group of patients is a reduced or absent palatal cingulum on the upper incisors. This can be another factor contributing to the excessive overbite. There is also an increased chance of the teeth being smaller than normal. Occasionally there is a reduced crown/root angulation, although beware the superimposition effect between central and lateral incisors on lateral cephalograms when making this diagnosis.

Oral health

Oral health is usually good, given a reasonable level of oral hygiene and dental care. In cases with excessive overbite, where the lower incisors occlude with the palatal mucosa and the upper incisors with the gingivae labial to the lower incisors, direct trauma to the gingivae may develop. This often does not arise until the patient reaches adult life, and it is much more common where there has been loss of posterior teeth. Where inflammation of the palatal mucosa associated with a deep, complete overbite is observed, the symptoms appear to be cyclical. Local oral hygiene is often an important factor in this presentation and should always be addressed first.

An excessive overbite is a potentially traumatic relationship; it should, where possible, be corrected in the early permanent dentition. This is not an easy correction and usually requires complex fixed appliance treatment.

Treatment aims

The main treatment aims can be summarized as follows:

1. To improve the aesthetics of the teeth and the function of the teeth and jaws but not at the expense of the lip and facial profile.
2. To relieve crowding and produce alignment of the teeth within the arches.
3. Where the overbite is excessive, to reduce it. Where the overbite is not excessively deep and there is tooth-to-tooth contact, it may then be best to accept the position of the upper central incisors and concentrate on alignment of the other teeth. If the overbite is to be reduced, the interincisal angle must also be reduced by torquing back the upper incisor apices with a fixed appliance.
4. If the overjet is increased, reduce it.

Treatment planning

It is of course essential to check that all teeth are present, sound and in favourable positions. The absence of third molars will not usually influence treatment unless extraction of second permanent molars is being considered. In fact this approach, or alternatively a non-extraction treatment, is not an uncommon choice in these cases, since space is provided by increasing the arch length when incisor inclinations are changed to improve the interincisal angle.

As is common in other malocclusions the planning process usually involves an initial assessment of the lower arch to estimate space requirements. As part of this process the crowding present, the overbite reduction necessary and the flattening of the curve of Spee that is required should all be considered in the calculation of the space needed for treatment.

In many cases a bimaxillary retroclination is an integral part of the presenting malocclusion. In order to obtain an improved profile and in the interests of obtaining a good finishing interincisal angle the incisors may, on occasion, be proclined during treatment. This procedure always carries a risk with regard to long-term stability but carries the best prognosis in Class II Division 2 malocclusions where incisors often present far more retroclined than normal.

The upper arch is examined from the point of view of crowding, torque requirements (where the upper incisors are significantly retroclined) and anchorage.

Treatment options

No treatment

In milder Class II Division 2 malocclusions in which the typical facial appearance is acceptable, as is the overbite, and the incisors are neither too retroclined nor too crowded, advising no active treatment can be a very reasonable approach to management.

Extractions only

This is rarely an acceptable treatment approach in this type of malocclusion. However, where buccal crowding is severe with a tendency for the premolars to be excluded from the arch this may be an option to consider, always provided that the Class II Division 2 pattern is mild.

Removable appliances

In these types of malocclusion an upper removable appliance is most frequently used to assist in the reduction of the deep overbite during the early stages of a fixed appliance treatment (adjunctive support). In a very limited number of cases a definitive simple removable treatment alone may be appropriate. An example might be where a labial spring is used to tuck a single proclined lateral incisor into the arch. This movement would be performed after an 'en masse' appliance (see Chapter 16) had been used to move the teeth of the buccal segments distally in a case where both the incisor alignment and overbite was otherwise acceptable.

The use of an isolated removable appliance, particularly in combination with a premolar extraction pattern, is rarely prescribed in Class II Division 2 malocclusion.

Single arch fixed appliances

An upper fixed appliance alone might be considered where the overbite and upper central incisor inclination is largely acceptable. Extra-oral traction might then be applied to the upper first molars via cemented fixed bands (see Chapter 17). When sufficient space has been achieved by this means or by a second premolar extraction when buccal segment crowding is present, an upper appliance may be fixed to the teeth to align and derotate the upper lateral incisors. Some limited torquing of incisor apices may be possible, as may limited centre-line corrections; otherwise these types of movement are best achieved with a full twin-arched fixed appliance.

Upper and lower arch fixed appliances

The vast majority of patients presenting with a Class II Division 2 malocclusion are best treated through the application of a full upper and lower fixed appliance.

Extraction pattern
The first option, which should always be considered, is whether this malocclusion may be corrected on the basis of 'no extractions' or alternatively loss of the permanent second molars. Often, where the incisors are retroclined, torquing the root apices palatally will increase the arch length and gain sufficient space to both align the dental arches and reduce the overbite. In such a situation a high level of patient compliance is essential since the end result depends on the extra-oral traction (headgear) being worn by the patient for long periods to supplement the anchorage. Where the incisors require more torque to achieve an acceptable interincisal angle, or there is a deeper initial overbite, or the crowding is more severe, then premolar extractions might be considered (usually four second premolars).

Occasionally, when only limited movements of lower teeth are deemed necessary, upper premolar extractions alone might be a valid plan in combination with a full fixed appliance. However, if this approach is to be taken a Class II molar relationship will result at the conclusion of treatment. There is some evidence that in such a circumstance, especially in Division 2 cases, that there is a higher risk of long-term lower incisor imbrication (and/or residual spacing in the upper arch) since the width of a premolar does not match half a molar.

Overbite
One of the chief reasons for employing a twin arch fixed appliance is to correct the overbite to a stable result. This is achieved by active intrusion of the lower incisors to flatten the curve of Spee. On occasions an upper removable appliance with an anterior bite plane may assist this process. In the upper arch where there is often an element of dento-alveolar vertical excess it is also desirable to intrude upper incisors; however, this movement is difficult to achieve consistently.

Interincisal angle
In many patients, by definition, the interincisal angle is obtuse at the start of treatment. Obtaining a stable overbite correction is dependent on torquing the incisor root apices palatally to achieve a more acute (reduced) interincisal angle, a solid 'occlusal stop' being formed by the incisor contact. Improving the incisor relationship in this way also improves the aesthetics and function of the finished occlusion.

The full fixed appliance is the most common, and reliable, approach to the treatment of mild to moderate Class II Division 2 malocclusions.

Functional appliances

Since some functional appliances are most effective in cases where the lower facial height is reduced their advocates have suggested their use in Class II Division 2 cases. The upper incisors are firstly proclined to create a Class II Division 1 malocclusion; this is then managed in the conventional manner (see Chapter 18). However, at least initially, the upper incisors are in a position of instability in relation to the lips (outside the area of soft tissue balance) and the functional appliance must be worn well to hold the upper incisor position whilst the created overjet is reduced.

Orthognathic surgery

In the more severe forms of this malocclusion, where the facial profile is poor and the overbite is very deep (and traumatic), a combination of orthodontics and jaw surgery is the best approach. Expert planning on the presentation of these types of severe malocclusion is important (see Chapter 22). In such cases in the initial presurgical phase of fixed appliance orthodontics, the upper incisors are proclined to create an overjet, whilst the deep overbite is maintained. The mandible is then advanced by surgery to reduce this overjet and correct the facial profile. Since the lower curve of Spee is maintained postsurgically there are lateral open bites. Subsequently these are closed orthodontically by extrusion of lower teeth of the buccal segments to preserve the increase in lower facial height gained in the surgery.

In only a limited number of Class II Division 2 cases is such a combined approach appropriate. Presurgical planning and orthodontics should only be undertaken by an appropriately skilled specialist team.

Post-treatment stability

Lateral incisor alignment

There is a very strong tendency for the lateral incisors to return part way towards their original position. This is particularly true if they were rotated. Where possible the position of these teeth should be overcorrected during treatment. Some authorities recommend prolonged retention but it is not yet clear whether retention beyond six months does improve stability or whether it merely postpones the relapse. As mentioned in Chapter 11, pericision is sometimes performed on these derotated teeth. Correction of these rotations early in any treatment is usually advisable. There is some evidence that these approaches reduce, even if they do not eliminate, relapse of rotations.

Overbites

As discussed earlier, relapse of overbite reduction will occur unless palatal movement of the incisor apices has reduced the interincisor angle. It is sometimes suggested that, in Class II Division 2 cases, proclination of upper and lower incisors (out of muscle balance) followed by permanent retention should be undertaken. The disadvantages of permanent retainers should not be overlooked: removable retainers will encourage food stagnation and plaque formation with consequent deterioration of the patient's oral health, and if they are left out even for a few weeks, relapse will occur. Fixed retainers are complex to make and need to be supervised very carefully.

However, there is no doubt that in some patients where there is considerable retroclination of the incisors the only feasible means of achieving an improved interincisal angle and full overbite correction involves allowing some forward movement of the incisors during the apical torquing process. Frequently, such a movement also complements the facial profile. It should be recognized that such movements, out of the classic position of muscle balance, should be undertaken with caution and the retention phase carefully supervised. Those cases where such a labial movement of the incisors is likely to remain stable are difficult to select with any degree of certainty.

Further reading

Mills, J.R.E. (1973). The problem of overbite in Class II Division 2 malocclusion. *British Journal of Orthodontics*, **1**, 34–8.

Williams, A. and Woodhouse, C. (1983). The crown root angle of maxillary incisors in different incisor classes. *British Journal of Orthodontics*, **10**, 159–61.

Chapter 14

Class III malocclusions

Class III malocclusion is found in about 3 to 5% of a Western population.

Occlusal and dento-alveolar features

According to Angle's classification, the lower arch should be at least one-half cusp width too far forward relative to the upper arch. Provided there is a Class III incisor relationship, the lower incisor tips lying anterior to the palatal cingulum of the upper incisors, milder degrees of prenormality are also included in this group of malocclusions (see Figure 7.4).

Labial segments

The upper incisors are often crowded and they are usually proclined. The lower incisors may be slightly crowded but they are often spaced. Frequently the lower incisors are retroclined. Thus, in many cases, the inclination of the incisors compensates to an extent for the underlying sagittal arch malrelationship. In other words there is usually dento-alveolar compensation of a Class III skeletal pattern.

By definition there is a Class III incisor relationship when the lower incisor edges are lying anterior to the cingulum plateau of the upper incisors. The lower incisors may lie anterior to the uppers so that there is a reverse overjet (see Figure 7.4) and an anterior displacement on closure may have contributed to this. The overbite varies considerably between cases. If there is incisor contact, the overbite will be reduced. Frequently if the anterior intermaxillary height is increased (and there is a large Frankfort– or maxillary–mandibular planes angle), there will be an anterior open bite (see Figure 10.1). Occasionally when there is a reverse overjet and the anterior intermaxillary height is low, the overbite will be deep.

Buccal segments

Frequently the upper arch is short antero-posteriorly so that the buccal segments are crowded: the canines may be mesially inclined and the first permanent molars distally inclined. In the developing occlusion, second and third molars may have become stacked and impacted (see Figure 9.1). Where there has been early loss of deciduous molar teeth, space reduction is rapid in the crowded

Mandibular positions and paths of closure

Usually there is a simple hinge closure from rest to occlusion. In a number of cases with a mild Class III incisor relationship and a normal or increased overbite, when the mandible is in centric relation, the incisors would meet edge-to-edge (with the posterior teeth out of occlusion) but, in order to obtain a position of maximal occlusion, there is a forward displacement of the mandible which exaggerates the severity of the occlusal and skeletal base malrelationship or discrepancy. A few of these cases may also overclose.

Where there is a unilateral crossbite with the teeth in occlusion there will usually be an associated lateral displacement of the mandible on closure. In theory, patients with occlusal disharmonies and mandibular displacements of the types described may be more liable to suffer from muscle pain, although there is limited evidence to support this contention. However, since it is straightforward, it usually makes sense to correct such displacements early as a simple interceptive measure. However, where the maxillary base is narrow and the inclination of the teeth already compensates for this to some extent, simple arch expansion may not be stable.

Soft tissues

Where the anterior intermaxillary height is large the lips are frequently incompetent. Such cases often have a skeletal anterior open bite, and during swallowing there will be an adaptive variation of swallowing behaviour with the tongue coming forwards into the gap between the incisors. Where the intermaxillary height is reduced sometimes the upper lip may also be shorter and hypotonic.

Growth

In most Class III cases it is usually best to proceed on the basis that any growth will be unfavourable, at least until this assumption is proved wrong!

This is due to the fact that dento-alveolar compensation is often at its limit by the time the patient enters their prepubertal growth spurt, the mandible grows more prognathic relative to the maxilla, and further dento-alveolar adaptation is not possible.

Where the height of the intermaxillary space is normal or reduced such growth may result in a worsening of the reverse overjet and the horizontal profile of the face.

Where the height of the intermaxillary space is increased with growth the tendency to a skeletal anterior open bite may become greater as the effect of the opening growth rotation (see Chapter 3) continues. Similarly, the growth tendency, in this case vertical, exceeds the limits of dento-alveolar adaptation and the anterior open bite may dramatically worsen with only posterior molars in contact. In such cases there is often a similarly dramatic effect on the vertical profile of the face.

Oral health

Mandibular displacements due to occlusal disharmonies eventually may be associated with muscle pain. Although it should be stressed that this could be only one factor out of many contributing to a presentation of temporomandibular joint pain dysfunction syndrome.

Where there is a premature contact in the incisor region there may be gingival recession around one or more lower incisors, but this is more common in Class I cases with a single instanding upper central incisor and an associated anterior displacement. Although in cases where there is an anterior open bite, periodontal changes might be expected around the non-functional teeth (those out of occlusion), no characteristic problems are found.

Treatment aims

The principal treatment aims can be summarized as follows:

1. To improve the aesthetics of the teeth and the function of the teeth and jaws whilst maintaining or improving the facial profile.
2. To relieve crowding and produce alignment within the arches.
3. To correct the incisor relationship to obtain a more normal overjet, overbite and interincisal angle.
4. To eliminate antero-posterior and unilateral lateral crossbites together with associated displacements.

Treatment planning

When treatment planning a Class III case it is important to establish the true occlusal position after all displacements have been eliminated. It is often of value to have two sets of records, one with the occlusion in the displaced position and the other set at the retruded condylar position with displacements eliminated. The patient will often present complaining of upper arch (canine) crowding associated with a narrow and/or short dental arch. In such cases the crowding should not be relieved without some consideration being given to the likely effect of future growth on the dental arch relationship. It is wise to develop a longer-term provisional treatment plan before arranging extraction of any permanent teeth.

Treatment options

No treatment

Where crowding of the dental arches is minimal, there are no displacements apparent, and the Class III appearance of the incisors and/or the jaws is acceptable, the 'no-treatment' option is a reasonable approach to management. It also has the advantages of keeping the Class III growth tendency under review and minimizing any intervention until growth has largely finished and the jaw profile has been finally established.

Extractions only

In many cases where the lower arch is well aligned, the upper arch is crowded, there is no displacement and the appearance of the Class III incisor and jaw discrepancy is acceptable to the patient; upper arch extractions only may appear a simple and attractive treatment. Usually upper first premolar loss is considered to facilitate the alignment of buccally excluded upper permanent canines, always provided that they are favourably (mesially) inclined.

Great care should be taken with this approach, since upper incisors can drop back into any residual extraction space, to worsen the incisor pattern. However, on occasions it is appropriate, although an upper removable space maintainer may, in addition to its usual role, act to support the position of the labial segment.

Removable appliance

Treatment with an upper removable appliance works particularly well where one or two incisors are 'caught behind the bite' and there is an associated forward displacement of the lower jaw. Such an approach is most frequently employed as an interceptive measure in the mixed dentition. An adequate overbite is essential at the completion of tooth movement to maintain the correction.

Occasionally a removable appliance may be used in company with a fixed appliance to clear the occlusion during the early stages of treatment or alternatively to provide an intermittent anchor in the lower arch from which to attach Class III intermaxillary elastics to an upper fixed appliance.

Single arch fixed appliance

An upper single arch fixed appliance may be considered when the lower is well aligned the jaw and incisor discrepancy is acceptable to the patient. In addition there should be no displacement but there are substantial rotations in the maxillary arch. Depending on the crowding, either first or second premolars would often be extracted.

Full arch fixed appliance

This would be the usual orthodontic approach to a purely dento-alveolar correction of this type of malocclusion. Before prescribing such an appliance a careful assessment is required. The underlying skeletal discrepancy should be relatively mild and susceptible to dento-alveolar camouflage, otherwise surgery will be necessary to achieve a correction. Ideally the upper incisors should at presentation be upright or retroclined and the lowers proclined, such that they may be tipped to make the correction. It is an advantage if there is also an initial anterior displacement on closure. The patient should be checked to see if they can obtain an edge-to-edge incisor contact; this is often indicative of a good prognosis for treatment providing that the incisal inclinations are favourable.

Before starting such treatment due consideration should be given to the pattern of growth since if this is unfavourable it could rapidly outstrip the amount of dento-alveolar movement available to disguise the underlying horizontal skeletal discrepancy.

In patients with a tendency towards an increased lower facial height, special care should be taken since most tooth movements in this type of case will tend to open the bite on the molars and encourage a further increase in the anterior intermaxillary height. This is especially true when upper arch expansion devices are employed (see Chapter 17). In patients with this type of tendency (towards an anterior open bite), growth modification may be possible by means of a high pull headgear to the upper first permanent molars. Such an approach is very dependent on active growth and good patient cooperation.

Extraction pattern
This will of course depend on the amount of horizontal movement of the incisors required and the degree of crowding present. In a typical case where upper incisors are to be tipped forwards (thus adding space to the arch) and the lower incisors are to be tipped back, a common extraction pattern might be removal of upper second premolars and lower first premolars.

Overbite
It is usually important to finish treatment with a positive overbite in order to maintain the incisor correction.

Interincisal angle
This should be within normal limits at the conclusion of treatment. If upper incisors are proclined too far or the lowers over-retroclined not only may the result be unstable but also the health of the supporting tissues may be prejudiced. In particular, transverse loading of an upper incisor can result in rapid periodontal breakdown.

In a suitable case a full fixed appliance can give an excellent and consistent result. However, case selection is particularly important in Class III cases. If dento-alveolar camouflage is attempted in a patient with a strongly active unfavourable growth pattern not only will treatment fail but future skeletal correction employing surgery may have been prejudiced also.

Functional appliance

This has been a popular treatment approach in Class III malocclusion in the past, the Frankel Fr. 3 (see Chapter 18) being a commonly used appliance. Usually, such an appliance was fitted early in the mixed dentition stage of occlusal development. Problems with the long-term retention of the occlusal result during continuing growth, and the essentially dento-alveolar nature of the correction have made such functional appliances less popular in contemporary orthodontic management of Class III malocclusion.

Orthognathic surgery

This has become increasingly popular in the treatment of patients with moderate to severe Class III skeletal discrepancy. An initial orthodontic phase is usually necessary in these patients to decompensate the arches by putting the teeth in the ideal positions to facilitate the surgery. The maxilla may be advanced or the mandible pushed back as the patient's profile and occlusion demands. Often a combination of upper and lower jaw surgery is necessary with the addition of a reduction genioplasty of the chin.

Vertical skeletal excess may be dealt with by the addition of a Le Fort 1 posterior impaction osteotomy. This is a commonly employed approach to the problem of skeletal anterior open bite. A more detailed description of surgical correction of Class III malocclusions is given in Chapter 22.

Over the last decade surgical correction has become a common approach to patients with significant Class III jaw and/or facial profile discrepancies. Approximately 30–40 per cent of patients presenting with a Class III might be suitable to consider a surgical correction. If a young patient shows early signs of developing such a problem and there is a chance of further unfavourable growth, dento-alveolar camouflage generally should be avoided. Such untimely interventions can create problems later if orthognathic correction is to be considered.

Surgery in these cases would usually be performed when all growth has ceased since otherwise there is a danger of the skeletal discrepancy regrowing.

Post-treatment stability

Stability of overjet correction depends in the short term on an adequate overbite and in the long term on facial growth. The greater part of orthodontic treatment is undertaken in the growing patient. On average, the mandible grows downwards and forwards slightly faster than the maxilla. In Class III patients this is an adverse growth trend and may result both in a worsening (or relapse) of the overjet and a reduction in overbite. An early sign of this happening is loss of overbite on the upper lateral incisors with the result that they relapse into a reverse overjet.

In some patients the Class III skeletal pattern will become markedly more severe after treatment and in these cases relapse is inevitable. In other patients the facial proportions change little during the later stages of growth and no adverse occlusal changes should result. In Class III, more than in other types of malocclusion, long-term stability depends on a favourable growth pattern, and this holds true whatever treatment approach is adopted.

Chapter 15

Tissue changes associated with tooth movement

The arrangement by which a tooth is suspended in a socket in the alveolar bone via the periodontal ligament is well known.

Normal alveolar bone

This consists of a layer of lamellated compact bone adjacent to both the periodontal membrane (lamina dura) and the oral mucosa. Cancellous or spongy bone is found between these two compact layers. The lamellae of the compact bone run parallel to the long axis of the tooth. On the labial or buccal sides of the alveolar crest the bone is almost entirely compact.

The physical properties of bone situated elsewhere in the body and the reaction of this bone to different stresses is relatively well understood. However, this is not necessarily the case when examining those bony changes in the alveolus that occur in relation to stress associated with tooth loading.

Periodontal ligament

In general much less is known of the properties of the periodontal ligament (PDL) than those of bone. Histologically, it consists of collagenous connective tissue, cells, blood vessels and tissue fluids; additionally, it would appear to be viscoelastic although, apart from this, the physical properties are poorly defined. However, it would seem that as well as cushioning the tooth against sudden blows, having a role in eruption and mediating sensory response, this ligament is also vital in the process of orthodontic tooth movement.

The classic experiments on tissue changes following orthodontic loading and initial tooth movement were performed by Sandstedt and by Oppenheim, first on monkeys and then on humans early in the 1900s. Much of our understanding of tooth movement is still based on these early studies together with later work by Reitan in the 1960s and 1970s on the tissue response of the PDL, bone and cementum to load.

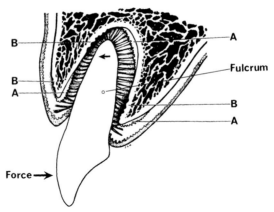

Figure 15.1 The effects of a tipping force: A, areas of bone deposition; B, areas of bone resorption

Types of tooth movement

Tipping (Figure 15.1)

This is produced typically by application of a single point force via a removable orthodontic appliance. With light forces the fulcrum is about 40% of the length of the root from the apex.

Bodily movement and rotation

Usually, these are not practicable with removable appliances since they require the application of a force couple. However, most fixed appliances are capable of producing bodily tooth movements and rotations through their potential to transport both crown and root through three dimensions of space.

Extrusion and intrusion

The force distribution within the periodontal ligament depends on the nature of the tooth movement. With tipping movements, areas of maximal pressure and tension are set up at the apical and cervical regions of the root, whereas with bodily movements the force is distributed reasonably evenly along the root axis. Extrusion and intrusion of teeth are also possible, although much reduced forces are required in the latter instance since the force is being concentrated at the small apical area of the root.

Tissue changes

The tissue changes produced depend principally on the values and duration of the forces used. Different regions of the periodontal ligament may show different types of tissue reaction at any one time depending on the force values within the periodontium at that particular point.

Within the first 24 hours after the application of the force, the tooth moves some way through the periodontal space, setting up areas of tension and compression within the periodontium. This initial movement appears to be, at least in part, a viscoelastic effect.

Areas of pressure

Light forces

Light forces are typically 30 g or 0.03 N per single-rooted tooth for tipping movement. The periodontal ligament is compressed but not crushed and the blood vessels remain patent. Within 24–48 hours osteoclasts appear along the bone surface and direct bone resorption proceeds. Within the cancellous spaces, deposition of osteoid takes place.

Heavy forces

The periodontal ligament is crushed between the tooth and the socket wall. The blood vessels are occluded and the periodontal ligament becomes acellular and hyaline in appearance. The osteocytes of the underlying bone die. These hyalinized areas are often fairly localized, and osteocytes appear adjacent to them and within the cancellous spaces of the underlying bone. In this manner the hyalinized area is removed by undermining resorption and the tooth will eventually move. If the range of action of the force (e.g. spring) has been large, the force applied will still be excessive and further areas of hyalinization will appear.

Areas of tension

Initially there is a proliferation of fibroblasts and preosteoblasts and the periodontal fibres are elongated. Osteoid tissue is deposited along the bone surface in spicules, lying in the direction of the stretched periodontal fibres. Subsequently this osteoid tissue is progressively replaced by bundle bone.

Where heavy forces have been used, the periodontal fibres on the tension side may be torn and blood vessels ruptured. When the tooth is being moved labially or palatally, modelling resorption and deposition on the external alveolar surface, particularly in the marginal region, will maintain the thickness and contour of the alveolar plates.

Retention

Retention is the term applied to that period of treatment during which the teeth are held passively after orthodontic correction has been achieved (see Chapter 25). During the period of retention further tissue changes take place. In the tension areas the remaining osteoid is replaced by bundle bone, which in turn is reorganized to form lamellated bone with Haversian systems.

In the regions of pressure the osteoclasts remain for up to two weeks. Osteoid is deposited over the areas of resorption and, in due course, this is replaced by bundle bone and ultimately by mature lamellated bone.

The periodontal fibres also become reorganized during the retention period. Most of these changes are completed within six months. However, reorganization

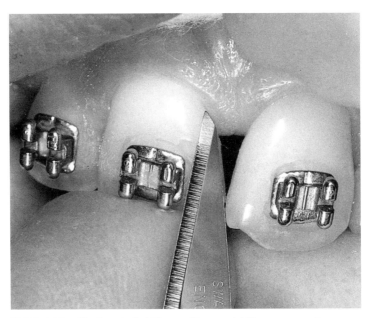

Figure 15.2 Pericision. The free gingival fibres and trans-septal fibres are severed

is much slower after certain tooth movements; for example, after rotations, the trans-septal and free (circum-) gingival fibres remain displaced for a considerable time. It is possible that the failure of readaptation of these fibres contributes towards relapse of such tooth movements. For this reason, surgical section or pericision (Figure 15.2) of these fibres may be undertaken following tooth alignment. This does not always eliminate relapse but appears to be effective in reducing the relapse tendency provided that it is correctly performed. The tooth should then be retained in the conventional manner for about six to nine months. Another approach to this problem is to correct any tooth rotations early in the active treatment phase; they are then effectively retained throughout appliance therapy.

Force and tissue change: the contemporary view

The preceding description of tissue change in reaction to a force on a tooth was first described nearly 40 years ago. However, the precise mechanism by which stresses are set up within the periodontal ligament and how such stresses mediate cellular change with resultant orthodontic tooth movement is still not understood. Computer models employing sophisticated finite element stress analysis software, as previously applied to bridge and building design in engineering, have been used to define these stresses together with the resultant strains. Such a three-dimensional model (Figures 15.3 and 15.4) confirms the basic, if simplistic, description given previously (Figure 15.1) but it also demonstrates that the arrangement of stresses in the ligament is constantly changing, in both magnitude and direction. This holds true even in the scenario of a steady single point load applied to a single-rooted tooth.

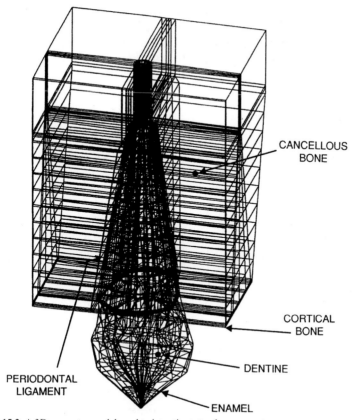

Figure 15.3 A 3D computer model used to investigate tooth movement

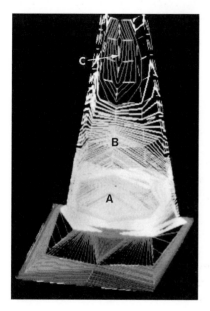

Figure 15.4 The complicated pattern of stresses in the periodontal ligament: A, compression; B, intermediate; C, tension. Viewed from the direction in which the tooth is moving

This more recent type of study has also indicated that, although the traditional view of a single-rooted tooth tipping about a point 40% from the apex makes sense in a two-dimensional diagram, in the true situation where one is operating in three dimensions the picture is more complicated. The centre of rotation appears to move constantly within an elliptical area towards the apical third of the root (see McGuinness *et al.*, 1992).

The factors linking stress to cellular response are also largely unknown although piezoelectric and various chemical factors (e.g. prostaglandins) have been implicated (Sandy and Harris, 1984).

This lack of detailed knowledge on how teeth move goes someway to explaining the unpredictability of individual tooth responses in the clinical situation. One reason for this difference in individual response is the variation in the physical properties of the periodontal ligament with relation to age and disease. Both of these factors have been demonstrated to affect the strain response and thus ultimately cause a varied resultant tooth movement. This is one of the reasons why orthodontic treatment in the adult (over 16 years) is different and is considered separately in Chapter 21.

Force magnitude

The threshold value below which tooth movement will not occur is very low. For tipping movements a very light force should be applied initially and this can be increased to about 30–70 g (0.03–0.07 N) for a single-rooted tooth. The force applied should be proportional to the root area and correspondingly heavier forces may be applied to molar teeth.

Heavier forces may also be used for bodily tooth movement as the force is more evenly distributed throughout the periodontal ligament.

Shown below are possible ranges for force application to a typical single-rooted tooth. Larger forces may be appropriate where larger rooted teeth are to be moved, especially when in groups and when applied intermittently (to convert grams to Newtons multiply by 1000).

Tip = 30–70 g
Bodily = 100–150 g
Extrude = 30–100 g
Intrude = 10–30 g.

Rate of tooth movement

About 1 mm per month may be regarded as an acceptable rate of tooth movement. However, various factors, including the rate of growth and local tissue turnover, may affect the rate of tooth movement.

Nature and duration of the force applied

Both light and heavy forces will result in orthodontic tooth movement. However, it is generally felt that light continuous forces minimize hyalinization of the periodontal ligament, the rate of tooth movement being faster and more efficient. Heavier intermittently applied force is less likely to maintain a physiological tissue response.

The effect of age

In the adult, the periodontal ligament is much less cellular than in the child. In addition, the alveolar bone in children is less dense than in older patients. This means that, in general, tissue turnover and thus tooth movement will be slower in the adult patient, particularly in the early stages of treatment.

Individual variations

There is considerable individual variation in the response to orthodontic forces. This is at least in part dependent on the density of the alveolar bone. In some individuals the alveolar bone is cancellous with large marrow spaces, whereas in others it is dense lamellated bone with few marrow spaces. Tooth movement will be much slower in the latter.

Harmful effects of orthodontic tooth movement

Pulp death

This is not common but can result from the application of heavy forces, particularly if the apex of the tooth is closed. It is always wise to proceed cautiously where there is either evidence and/or a history of trauma to the tooth which it is planned to move. In such a situation the blood supply to the pulp may already have been prejudiced and the tooth may become discoloured and non-vital as the treatment progresses. This is not a common problem but when it occurs it is usually associated with an upper incisor.

Root resorption

Minor areas of resorption of cementum on the lateral aspects of the root may be seen during orthodontic tooth movement. These are not important and are usually repaired by cementum. Much more serious is the apical resorption sometimes seen, particularly when teeth have been moved bodily over long distances by fixed appliances. Such root damage may be extensive but little can be done. In severe cases some may advocate a calcium hydroxide dressing in the root canal to try to arrest the progress of the resorption. If such root resorption is observed during treatment the tooth movement should be stopped for some months to allow repair by secondary cementum and then, if absolutely neces-sary, tooth movement may be very carefully recommenced. It is important to recognize that root resorption is not uncommon in patients who have not received orthodontic treatment. For this reason all teeth to be moved should be radiographed prior to treatment.

Where evidence of *apical root blunting* or alternatively of *thin spindly roots* is seen on the initial radiographs, the clinician should be aware that these patients are more likely to experience root resorption during orthodontic treatment. If root resorption is observed, one should be very cautious about undertaking treatment and, if necessary, a regular clinical and radiographic review should be maintained during the period that the tooth is loaded.

General conclusions

It is generally thought that only light forces should be used for orthodontic tooth movement. Both vital and non-vital (endodontically treated) teeth can be moved.

Orthodontic movement is possible only because cementum is more resistant to resorption than bone. Some authors recommend intermittent pressure, others constant pressure. When properly applied, little clinical difference probably exists between the two approaches to treatment.

When excessive force is used it is very likely that the anchor teeth will move, the amount of force applied to them being ideal to encourage movement of larger rooted teeth. In such a situation the tooth that it is desired to move will often remain stationary due to the excessive force causing hyalinization of the ligament and local bone necrosis.

Further reading

Christiansen, R.L. and Burstone, C.J. (1969). Centres of rotation within the periodontal space. *American Journal of Orthodontics*, **55**, 353–69.

Davidovitch, Z., Finkelson, M.D., Steigman, S., *et al.* (1980). Electric currents, bone remodelling and orthodontic tooth movement. *American Journal of Orthodontics*, **77**, 33–47.

Jones, M.L., Hickman, J., Middleton, J. and Volp, C. (in press). A novel system for direct measurement of the PDL response to load in the human subject. *Journal of Orthodontics*, **28**, 24–30.

Jones, M.L., Middleton, J., Volp, C. *et al.* (1998). Biomechanical modelling in orthodontics – following a theme? The development of a validation system for FE modelling of tooth movement. In *Computer Methods in Biomechanics and Biomedical Engineering*, Book 2 (J. Middleton, M.L. Jones and G.N. Pande, eds) London: Gordon & Breach.

McGuinness, N.J.P., Wilson, A.N., Jones, M.L. and Middleton, J. (1992). A stress analysis of the periodontal ligament under various orthodontic loadings. *European Journal of Orthodontics*, **13**, 231–42.

Oppenheim, A. (1942). Human tissue response to orthodontic intervention of short and long duration. *American Journal of Orthodontics and Oral Surgery*, **28**, 263–301.

Proffit, W.R. (2000). The biologic basis of orthodontic therapy. In *Contemporary Orthodontics*, Chapter 9, pp. 296–325. St Louis: Mosby-Yearbook.

Reitan, K. (1960). Tissue behaviour during orthodontic tooth movement. *American Journal of Orthodontics*, **46**, 881–900.

Reitan, K. (1985). Biomechanical principles and reactions. In *Orthodontics: Current Principles and Technique*. (T.M. Graber and B.F. Swain, eds). St Louis: Mosby-Yearbook.

Rygh, P. (1989). The periodontal ligament under stress. In *The Biology of Orthodontic Tooth Movement*. Boca Raton, FL: CRC Press.

Sandy, J.R. and Harris, M. (1984). Prostaglandins and tooth movement. *European Journal of Orthodontics*, **6**, 175–82.

Wilson, A.N., McGuinness, N., Jones, M.L. and Middleton, J. (1991). A finite element study of canine retraction with a palatal spring. *British Journal of Orthodontics*, **18**, 211–18.

Yettram, A.L., Wright, K.W. and Houston, W.J.B. (1977). Centre of rotation of a maxillary central incisor under orthodontic loading. *British Journal of Orthodontics*, **4**, 23–7.

Yoshida, S., Tanne, K., Knox, J. and Jones, M.L. (1998). An evaluation of the biomechanical responses of tooth and periodontium to orthodontic forces in adolescent and adult subjects. *British Journal of Orthodontics*, **25**, 109–15.

Chapter 16

Removable appliances

Removable appliances are orthodontic devices that can be taken out of the mouth by the patient for cleaning. Myofunctional appliances are sometimes called removable appliances in North America (see Chapter 18).

Removable appliances have a limited role in modern orthodontics. They may be active or passive. Active appliances are chiefly confined to use in the mixed dentition, producing simple tipping tooth movements using wire springs or bows, screws, elastics or the acrylic baseplate. Passive appliances are designed to maintain teeth in their present position (e.g. space maintainers or retainers). The main components of a removable appliance are as follows:

1. Active component.
2. Retention (fixation).
3. Anchorage.
4. Baseplate.

Some of the components will have a dual function.

Active component

This provides the force that moves the tooth, which may be derived from wire springs or bows, screws or elastics.

Springs are made from hard stainless-steel wire. The simplest spring is the cantilever (Figure 16.1a).

The factors affecting the force (F) applied by this spring are given by the expression:

$$F \sim dr^4/l^3$$

In other words, the force is directly proportional to the deflection (d), to the fourth power of the radius (r) and inversely proportional to the cube of the length (l) of the wire. Thus, small variations in the length and particularly in the diameter of the wire will have major effects on the spring characteristics.

A light continuous force is considered to be the ideal force to produce optimum tooth movement (see Chapter 15). To achieve this the wire should be made as long as possible within the confines of the oral cavity and as thin as is consistent with adequate strength. Incorporating a coil (Figure 16.1b) may increase the effective length of the spring. For maximum stored energy

a

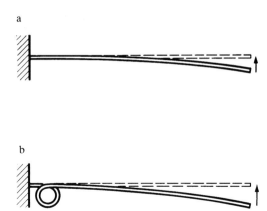

b

Figure 16.1 (a) A simple cantilever. (b) The incorporation of a coil increases the deflection of the spring for a given load. Note that the coil should unwind as the tooth moves

(i.e. resilience), the coil should unwind as the force is dissipated (Figure 16.1b). This is not always possible with buccal springs.

The spring must be carefully designed so that the tooth will move in the direction intended. The direction of movement is perpendicular to the tangent to the tooth surface at the point of contact of the spring (Figure 16.2). It is very common to find that palatal springs are placed too far back, so that the resultant force is buccally directed. Palatal finger springs are readily distorted and should be protected, either by being boxed within a recess of the baseplate or guarded by a length of wire or preferably both (Figure 16.3). The free action of the spring must not be impeded by the box or guards.

Labial bows are mechanically more complex than springs and their flexibility in the horizontal plane depends to a great extent on the height of any vertical loops incorporated in them. Supported bows, such as the Robert's retractor

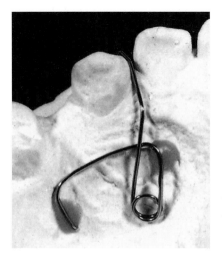

Figure 16.2 A palatal spring with a guard. This spring is positioned so that the tooth will be moved in the line of the arch: the tooth will move perpendicular to the tangent to the surface at the point of contact with the spring

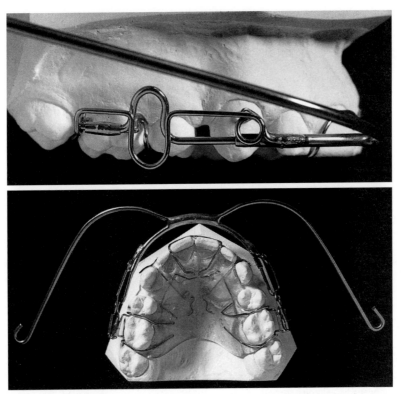

Figure 16.3 A simple appliance to retract upper canines with palatal springs. It is usually wise to have tubes attached to the clasps on the molars so that, if required, a facebow (the outer bow) can be fitted to them and anchorage can be reinforced by extra-oral traction worn in the evening and at nights. If a facebow was to be fitted for regular use to the appliance shown then an anterior clasp on the incisors and a locking catch should be included

(Figure 16.4), are made from 0.5 mm diameter wire. This bow, made from thinner wire, is very much more flexible, and mechanically advantageous.

Screws may be designed to act directly on the teeth through the baseplate (Figure 16.5). A screw applies a heavy intermittent force to the teeth, which is not considered to be ideal. In most cases screws should be activated, by the

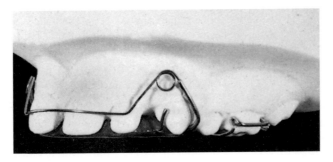

Figure 16.4 A Robert's retractor

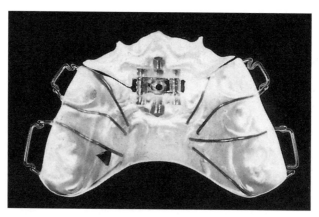

Figure 16.5 A screw plate to procline four upper incisors

patient, one quarter-turn each week. This opens the screw by about 0.2 mm. Thus the tooth movement is small and the periodontal ligament is not crushed. Weekly activation of the screw is usually appropriate. They may also be used to contract dental arches by constructing the appliance with the screw already opened. Screws have the disadvantages that compared with springs they are bulky and expensive.

Elastics are usually used as an aesthetic alternative to a wire bow for reduction of an overjet. They are not commonly used as the active component because they can slide up the labial surface of the teeth and damage the gingiva. Placement of elastics directly to teeth (to close a midline diastema, for instance) should not be carried out as this can lead to severe periodontal damage and possible loss of the teeth.

Fixation or retention

Retention is a term used to describe the means by which the appliance resists displacement. Retention is also used to describe the period following active tooth movement during which the teeth are held in their new positions while they stabilize (see Chapter 25). To avoid confusion the term fixation is preferable.

Fixation is usually provided by clasps or bows. Adequate fixation can be obtained from Adams clasps on the molars (Figure 16.6a) and, provided that the incisors are not being moved by springs, a Southend clasp on the central incisors (Figure 16.6b). Appliances with inadequate fixation will be unable to deliver the correct force to the tooth, will be uncomfortable for the patient and will encourage poor wear.

Remember that teeth to be moved should not have any form of fixation, unless a screw plate is being used, as the clasp will prevent movement. Adjustment of incisor positions in Class II Division 1 malocclusions is achieved by a labial bow, which will tend to provide its own fixation. Additional fixation can be obtained by clasping the canines. This has the advantage of preventing canines moving mesially, but the mesial arm of the clasp may occupy space that

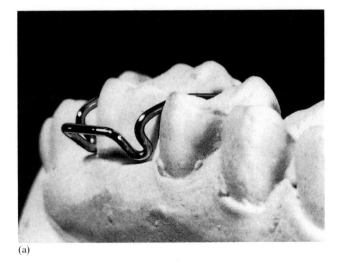

(a)

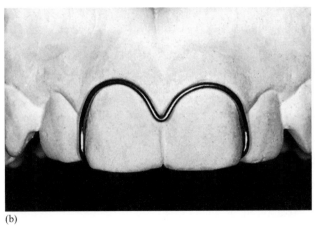

(b)

Figure 16.6 (a) An Adams clasp. Note the arrowhead engages in undercuts on the mesiobuccal and distobuccal aspects of the molar but does not contact the adjacent teeth. (b) A Southend clasp

is necessary for complete overjet reduction, and modification or removal of the clasp may be necessary in the later stages of treatment.

Anchorage

This is the resistance to the reactive forces generated by the active components of the appliance. Anchorage may be preserved by:

1. Placement of clasps or bows on teeth which are not being moved.
2. Contact of the baseplate with other teeth not being moved.
3. Contact of the baseplate with the vertical part of the palate in the area of the rugae (for distal movement of teeth).

4. Use of light forces to move teeth.
5. Movement of a single tooth per quadrant.
6. Intermaxillary elastics (see below).
7. Extra-oral traction – headgear (see below).

The resistance to tooth movement is related to:

1. The surface area of the roots.
2. The type of tooth movement permitted: teeth can be tipped more readily than they can be moved bodily. By designing the appliance so that the anchor teeth cannot tip, the anchorage is increased. However, although this is a common practice with fixed appliances, it is not easy with removable appliances.
3. Other factors, such as the intercuspation of the teeth may contribute to the anchorage.

For descriptive purposes, certain terms are used to classify the various forms of anchorage.

Intramaxillary is where the teeth within the same arch are used as anchorage. This anchorage may be:

- *Simple*, where teeth of greater resistance are used as anchorage for movement of a tooth or teeth of lesser resistance, for example pushing an incisor 'over the bite' against the buccal segment teeth.
- *Reciprocal*, where two teeth or groups of teeth of equal resistance are used to move each other reciprocally to an equal extent in opposite directions, for example transverse arch expansion.

Intermaxillary anchorage is where the opposing arch is used for anchorage. This anchorage may also be simple or reciprocal.

Intermaxillary anchorage is most commonly used with fixed appliances where elastics are stretched from the front of one arch to the back of the other (the direction of pull depending on the malocclusion to be treated). However, this is rarely used with removable appliances because the force of the elastics may overcome the fixation of the appliances.

Extra-oral anchorage may be used with a removable appliance, where a 'head cap' or 'neck strap' is used to provide, or reinforce, anchorage. When extra-oral anchorage is used as reinforcement to the intramaxillary anchorage, a removable 'facebow' is usually used to transmit the forces to the appliance. The headgear should be worn at night and the force applied should be about twice that provided by the active component of the appliance.

Where anchorage is entirely extra-oral and the force is applied by extra-oral elastics, as in the en masse appliance for retraction of upper buccal segments (Figure 16.7), the appliance need be worn only with the headgear. For an acceptable rate of progress, the headgear and appliance must be worn for more than 12 hours out of every 24. Many large-rooted teeth are being moved and so quite heavy forces are appropriate – up to 500 g (about 5 N) in all.

Safety: It is possible for J hooks or removable facebows to become disengaged, either during play or at night. A few cases have been reported of serious soft tissue laceration or even damage to an eye resulting in the loss of sight. Various types of safety headgear or safety straps are available to minimize the risk of this happening. These should be used routinely with J hooks or detachable

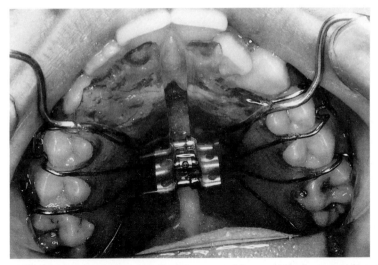

Figure 16.7 An 'en masse' appliance for distal movement of the upper buccal segments. Note the midline screw to expand the buccal teeth as they move distally, and Adams clasps on the first molars and premolars to assist retention (fixation)

facebows. To avoid problems of headgear detachment, it is good practice to either design the headgear as an integral part of the appliance or employ an extra-oral bow that locks (see Chapter 17).

Generally, extra-oral support for anchorage should only be employed by or under the supervision of an appropriately trained orthodontist.

Baseplate

This is usually made of cold-cure acrylic, which should only be as thick as is consistent with the strength required. This is quicker and more convenient to use than heat-cure acrylic. A heat-cure acrylic baseplate may be necessary for adults or children with a strong bite. Various coloured acrylics are available which can enhance acceptance of the appliance by the patient.

The baseplate performs the following functions:

1. Supports the wire or screw components.
2. Contributes to anchorage by contact with the palate and with teeth that are not to be moved.
3. Prevents unwanted drift of teeth.
4. Transmits forces from the active components to the anchorage.
5. Protects palatal springs.
6. May be extended to form anterior or posterior bite planes.

Anterior bite planes

These are used in order to reduce a deep overbite. They are also useful for relieving occlusal interference with tooth movement in cases with an initial deep

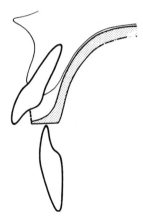

Figure 16.8 Trimming an anterior bite plane to allow incisor retraction. So that the lower incisors will still occlude with it, the bite plane should not be trimmed back too far. Then it is undermined to clear well away from the palatal surface of the upper incisors

overbite. Overbite reduction with an anterior bite plane depends largely on occlusal movement of the posterior teeth that are held out of occlusion, and some minor intrusion of the lower incisors. Anterior bite planes are usually successful in growing children who have an increased curve of Spee in the lower arch.

In Class II cases, overbite reduction should be commenced at the canine retraction stage. The bite plane should exceed the freeway space by 2–3 mm. When the incisors are retracted, a somewhat thicker plane should be constructed or a low plane may be thickened by addition of cold-cure acrylic (Figure 16.8). It is useful when designing an appliance to record the size of overjet so that the technician can extend the bite plane by an appropriate amount.

Posterior bite planes

These are used to clear occlusal interferences to tooth movement (particularly where there is a mandibular displacement) in appliances for correction of unilateral crossbite (Figure 16.9a) and instanding upper incisors (Figure 16.9b). For comfort, the occlusal coverage of the posterior teeth should be only just thick enough to clear the occlusion.

Construction of removable appliances

Materials used

Stainless steel
In orthodontic work, 18:8 hard austenitic stainless-steel wire is used.

- *Advantages.* Cheap, strong, resilient, not affected by the oral fluids, and fairly easy to manipulate, and may be easily welded. (The pieces to be welded are held together under pressure and a current is passed. The resistance at the junction of the parts results in a rise in temperature and fusion occurs due to localized melting at the point of juncture. The grain structure of the wire should not be seriously affected. A high-density low-voltage current is used (100 A, 5 V) and the time of the weld is made very brief (0.01 s) to avoid overheating of the wire adjacent to the weld.)

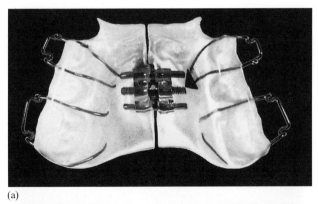

(a)

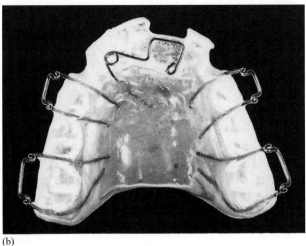

(b)

Figure 16.9 (a) An appliance to expand the upper arch. Acrylic covering the occlusal surfaces of the premolars and molars will relieve any cuspal interference from the lower teeth, which may hinder tooth movement. (b) An appliance to procline an instanding incisor with a palatal finger spring. Note that it is cranked to avoid contact with the other incisors and protected by an acrylic cover. Acrylic covering the premolars and molars will prop the bite open and prevent the incisal overbite from hindering tooth movement

- *Disadvantages.* Must be worked in hard state, but excessive working causes fatigue and fracture. Soldering is difficult and requires special flux, and even then union is poor. Special fluoride-containing fluxes are necessary to remove the passive surface film of chromium oxide. A low-fusing silver solder is most suitable. The essential points to be observed are that the wires should be thoroughly cleaned, in close contact and liberally coated with flux. The area of the joint must be adequately heated using a gentle blue flame. The operation should be completed as rapidly as possible to minimize overheating and annealing the adjacent wire.

Acrylic resin
This is used for the baseplate.

Construction

Construction of removable appliances is carried out in the orthodontic laboratory to the prescription of the clinician. The instructions should be clear and unambiguous and the clinician should state what he or she wants the appliance to achieve. The design should be simple and should not carry too many active components. In addition to a written prescription, a drawing may also be helpful for the technician.

- *Adams clasps* are constructed from 0.7 mm diameter hard stainless-steel wire (HSSW) for all except deciduous teeth, where 0.5 mm diameter HSSW may be used instead.
- *Southend clasps* are constructed from heat-treated 0.7 mm diameter blue Elgiloy® wire.
- *Palatally approaching springs* which are protected by the baseplate are constructed from 0.5 mm diameter HSSW, or 0.7 mm diameter HSSW for molars.
- *Buccally approaching springs* may be *self-supporting*, in which case they are constructed from 0.7 mm HSSW. *Supported buccally approaching springs* are constructed from 0.5 mm HSSW, which is sheathed from the baseplate to the coil by 0.5 mm internal diameter stainless-steel tubing.

An example of a laboratory prescription card for an appliance to be used in the first stage of the correction of a Class II Division 1 malocclusion, with no anticipated anchorage problems and with the left canine buccally placed and the right canine in arch line, is shown in Figure 16.10.

For details of construction of the various components see Adams and Kerr (1990).

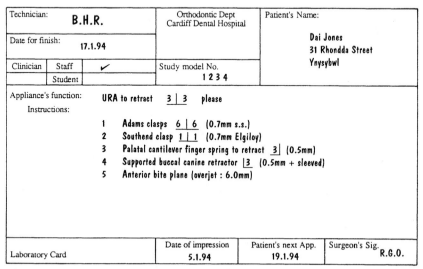

Figure 16.10 A laboratory card for an appliance to retract maxillary canines. The right canine is in arch line, but the left canine is buccally placed and therefore needs a buccally approaching spring to correct its position. Note that the patient has a Class II Division 1 malocclusion, and an anterior biting platform has been incorporated into the design to reduce an increased overbite. A second appliance will be necessary to reduce the overjet

Indications for removable appliances

The key to all successful orthodontic treatment is a correct diagnosis and treatment plan. When used under the correct circumstances and in competent hands, treatment using removable appliances can provide a simple and economic solution to occlusal problems. Removable appliances are capable of:

- simple tipping movements
- overbite reduction
- elimination of occlusal interferences
- space maintenance/retention
- minor derotations of incisor teeth
- simple extrusion in conjunction with a fixed attachment.

A typical example of an appliance to tip teeth both distally and palatally is shown in Figure 16.4. If a tooth is to be tipped, its initial position must be with excessive tip so that, in its final position, it is ideally angled with a mild mesial tip, although an upright position is acceptable. A tooth should not finish with its crown distal to the root, as it will suffer inappropriate load on the periodontal ligament, which will be non-physiological (pathological) during function.

It should be remembered that proclination of a tooth to correct an incisor crossbite will effectively reduce the overbite, and a positive overbite at the end of treatment is essential for stability. Conversely, retroclination of an incisor to correct an increased overjet will effectively increase the overbite, and will require overbite control to allow a Class I incisor relationship to be established.

Elimination of occlusal interferences

Anterior or posterior bite planes will efficiently eliminate occlusal interferences, which may hinder crossbite correction. Lower removable appliances with bite planes may also be used to assist a maxillary fixed appliance, which is attempting crossbite correction.

Space maintenance/retention

Keeping space in the dental arch for unerupted teeth can be achieved by a variety of means. The advantage of a removable appliance for this purpose is that it can incorporate an anterior bite plane to control the overbite. It is also easy to attach a prosthetic tooth to the baseplate. The tooth will not only act as a space maintainer, but also provide an occlusal stop for opposing teeth and, in cases with an absent anterior tooth, enhance aesthetics. A passive removable appliance is frequently used as a retainer following active tooth movement.

Minor derotations of incisor teeth

A force couple, i.e. two wires acting in opposite directions on diametrically opposed corners of the incisor tooth, will cause derotation (Figure 16.11a). This is only possible if the rotated tooth is upright. Careful adjustment of the appliance is needed to achieve a satisfactory result. Remember that a rotated incisor occupies less space in the arch, and space will be required for derotation.

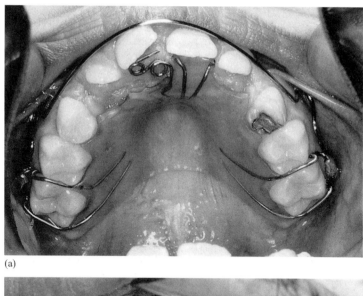

(a)

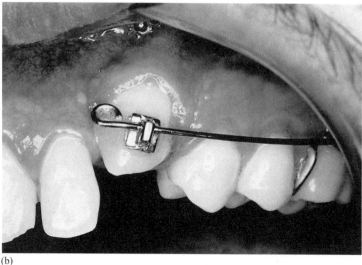

(b)

Figure 16.11 (a) A force couple acting on a rotated central incisor. The palatal 'Z' spring is active on the distopalatal corner and the labial bow is active on the mesiolabial corner of the crown of the tooth. (b) Extrusion of a maxillary canine using a combination of a fixed and removable appliance in an adult. A Begg bracket has been directly bonded onto the labial surface of the crown, and a free-ended wire spur in 0.6 mm hard stainless-steel wire has been soldered onto the Adams clasp on the first molar. The spur is adjusted to lie just below the level of the incisal edge of the lateral incisor, and is lifted up and placed in the vertical slot of the Begg bracket. This tooth was successfully moved in three months

Simple extrusion of teeth in conjunction with a fixed attachment

The wide palatal coverage of a removable appliance provides excellent anchorage. This can be particularly helpful when straightforward vertical movement of a tooth is necessary, such as extrusion of a partially erupted maxillary canine, or an incisor with a fracture that needs extrusion to simplify restorative care. A free-ended spring, with a coil for additional flexibility, constructed in 0.5 mm HSSW, hooks over a suitable attachment on the tooth (Figure 16.11b).

Fitting removable appliances

There are several steps involved in fitting an appliance:

1. Before the patient arrives:
   (a) Check that you have the correct appliance for the patient.
   (b) Check that the appliance matches the laboratory prescription.
   (c) Check the fit surface of the appliance has no sharp projections (it is often easier to detect these without gloves).
   (d) Check that the appliance fits the model and that the time since the date of the impression is not unacceptably long.
   (e) Check the positioning of the components.
   (f) Check that there is free movement of the active components.
   (g) Check that the headgear bow is a rigid and tight fit to the tubes in the appliance. If there is a locking mechanism (the preferred option), check that it works.
2. With the patient:
   (a) Check the fit of the appliance.
   (b) Check and adjust the extension of the baseplate, e.g. trim acrylic from the path of teeth to be moved.
   (c) Adjust the active components.
   (d) Adjust the retentive components.
   (e) Add and adjust headgear if necessary.
   (f) Take tooth position measurements, e.g. for retraction of canines measure distance between two reproducible points such as the cusp tip of the canine and the mid-buccal groove of the first molar. Impaling the patient's file with the points of the dividers obviates the need to record the distance in millimetres. Record which landmarks have been chosen. This can be repeated at subsequent visits and comparison made to check progress. Measure overjet (with appliance out of the mouth) and record in the patient's file.
   (g) Ask patient if appliance feels comfortable. N.B. If this is the patient's first appliance it will feel strange and a real 'mouthful', but it should not be uncomfortable.
   (h) Demonstrate insertion and removal of the appliance with the components in their correct positions to both the patient and parent (if appropriate).
   (i) Check that patient can achieve insertion and removal unaided.
   (j) Give instructions on hours of wear (almost always full-time wear) and cleaning (toothbrush and toothpaste at least once a day). Issue wear chart if necessary. Back up verbal instructions with a written sheet.
   (k) Warn patient of initial difficulties in acclimatizing to the appliance, e.g. eating and speaking, and reassure that after 48 hours or so these difficulties will ameliorate. Ask if there are any questions about appliance.
   (l) Give subsequent appointment; this will usually be in four weeks' time.
3. At the subsequent visit:
   (a) Ask patient and/or parent about any difficulties with appliance.

(b) Ask patient about wear of appliance. Often the wear of the appliance is dictated by difficulties experienced. If a headgear is fitted, check fit and make sure it does not become detached at night.

(c) Adjust appliance to overcome reported difficulties if necessary.

(d) Repeat measurements to check tooth movement. Between 1 and 2 mm per month movement is satisfactory progress. Untoward overjet increase when moving buccal teeth distally indicates loss of anchorage. See above for methods of preserving anchorage.

(e) Check condition of mouth. Look for marginal gingivitis especially on the palatal aspects adjacent to the baseplate, trauma from the baseplate, retentive or active components and candidal infection beneath the baseplate. Give appropriate advice, prescription or adjustment of appliance.

(f) Reactivate components or, if the tooth movements that the appliance was designed to achieve are complete, then stop treatment or take an impression for the next appliance. Remember at this stage to keep the current appliance passive so that the new appliance will fit.

(g) Tell patient (and parent) of progress, or lack of progress.

(h) Give subsequent appointment.

Appliance not being worn

There are several signs which can indicate that the appliance is not being worn:

1. There is little or no tooth movement.
2. The appliance still looks new. The baseplate retains its high polish, and does not become cloudy due to absorption of oral fluids.
3. The patient's speech is affected when the appliance is in the mouth.
4. The patient has difficulty removing and, more importantly, inserting the appliance.
5. The springs are still active.
6. The appliance may not fit well, as there may have been tooth movement when the appliance was out of the mouth.
7. There will be no imprint of the arrowhead of the Adams clasp on the gingivae.
8. There will be no outline of the shape of the baseplate on the palate.
9. The patient may admit to not wearing the appliance. Possible reasons for this include:
   (a) instructions misunderstood
   (b) pain or discomfort
   (c) appliance broken/lost
   (d) appearance
   (e) dislike/intolerance of appliance.

The clinician should identify the cause for lack of wear and attend to the problem. It is important that both patient and parent realize the importance of compliance with appliance wear.

Unsuccessful appliance therapy

This may be due to poor compliance (see above), iatrogenic factors and intrinsic patient factors.

Iatrogenic factors

- Incorrect choice of treatment mechanics, i.e. attempting to correct a malocclusion using the wrong type of appliance.
- Incorrect choice of extractions. This usually means extraction of second premolars rather than first premolars and having insufficient space to achieve full alignment. The reverse can also be true, with too much space being left at the end of treatment.
- Poor anchorage control.
- Incorrect appliance design. Although a removable appliance might be suitable for correction of the malocclusion, incorrect design will hinder progress.
- Poor fit of appliance, leading to patient discomfort. May be due to overlong period between taking impression and fitting appliance. This problem of fit may be compounded if extractions have been performed in the interim. Normally a removable appliance should be fitted within 1 month of taking the impression, and preferably sooner if extractions have been carried out.
- Baseplate trimmed incorrectly. Failure to clear acrylic from the path of the advancing tooth, or to appreciate the bunching-up of soft tissues in front of the tooth can prevent tooth movement.
- Too many active components. The appliance should be designed to move only a small number of teeth. It is preferable to use two or more appliances to achieve correction than to try incorporating all the components into one appliance.
- Active components incorrectly adjusted. Too much activation of springs, etc., is likely to cause loss of anchorage because the reaction to the heavy force on the tooth to be moved will be a light (optimal) force on the anchor teeth, encouraging their movement (see Chapter 15).
- Fixation (retentive) components ineffective. This will allow displacement of the appliance with a reduction in efficiency of the spring and will be uncomfortable for the patient.
- Trauma. Incorrectly placed or adjusted springs can cause trauma, which, in turn, will discourage appliance wear.
- Wrong instructions given to the patient regarding appliance wear.
- Unstable end-point of treatment. If the teeth have been moved into an unstable position there will, without permanent retention, always be relapse.

Intrinsic patient factors

In spite of a correctly designed, constructed, adjusted and worn appliance, teeth may still fail to move. This may be because the tooth is ankylosed, for example a previously traumatized incisor that has healed by ankylosis. There is nothing that can be done to move this tooth. There may be an area of sclerotic bone in the path of the tooth. This may be the result of a difficult extraction.

There may be anatomical limitations. Teeth can only be moved where there is bone. Severe skeletal discrepancies will require a combination of surgery and orthodontics to overcome these problems (see Chapter 22). At a local level, loss of alveolar bone will lead to a narrowing of the channel of cancellous bone through which the tooth can move easily.

Further reading

Adams, C.P. and Kerr, W.J.S. (1990). *The Design and Use of Removable Appliances*, 6th edn. Oxford: Butterworth-Heinemann.

Houston, W.J.B. and Walters, N.R.E. (1977). The design of buccal canine retraction springs for removable orthodontic appliances. *British Journal of Orthodontics*, **4**, 191–5.

Muir, J.D. and Reed, R.T. (1979). *Tooth Movements with Removable Appliances*. London: Pitman Medical.

Chapter 17

Treatment with fixed appliances

Fixed appliances are powerful and complex mechanisms and their unskilled use may lead to extensive and rapid unwanted tooth movements. The dental practitioner without special training should not attempt to use fixed appliances. However, he may need to refer patients requiring fixed appliance treatment to an orthodontic specialist. Thus he should have some knowledge of their scope and action.

Definition. A fixed appliance is an orthodontic device where attachments are fixed to the teeth. Forces are applied to the teeth via the action of arch wires or auxiliaries through these attachments. This allows precise three-dimensional control over the nature and direction of the forces applied.

Components of fixed appliances

Attachments

The attachments (brackets, tubes, etc.) are peculiar to each fixed appliance technique. Their function is to allow a controlled force (or a force 'couple') to be applied to the tooth (Figure 17.1). The attachments may be directly fixed to the teeth by means of etch-retained composite resin (Figure 17.2) or some similar system. Alternatively, the attachment may be welded to stainless-steel bands which are then, in turn, cemented to the teeth. Bands may be purchased in a variety of stock sizes or may be individually constructed from stainless-steel tape for teeth of unusual size or shape. Directly bonded attachments are

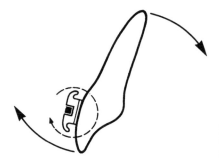

Figure 17.1 A mechanical couple can be applied to a tooth with a fixed appliance. This means that precise control over root movement is possible

Auxiliaries

Forces may be applied to the teeth by auxiliary springs or elastics. As an example, latex elastics are used for transmitting forces between the arches (intermaxillary traction) as well as within any one arch (intramaxillary traction).

Advantages and disadvantages of fixed compared with removable appliances

Fixed

1. Precise control over force distribution to individual teeth means that rotation and controlled root movement are possible.
2. Multiple tooth movements can be performed simultaneously.
3. Complex to make and use so special training is needed.
4. Chairside time is comparatively long.
5. Components are usually more costly (this is now less of a problem).
6. Oral hygiene is made more difficult.

Removable

1. Single point application of forces means that only tipping movements are readily produced.
2. Usually only a few teeth should be moved at any one time. The appliance should be kept as simple as possible.
3. Treatment should be kept comparatively simple and should be within the scope of the dental practitioner.
4. Only suitable for carefully selected cases.
5. Chairside time is usually short but laboratory time is generally greater than for fixed appliances.
6. Components are usually inexpensive and easy to obtain.
7. Since the appliance is removable the problems of oral hygiene should not be any greater than normal.

Limitations of fixed appliances

It should be recognized that many of the limitations of removable appliance treatment apply equally to fixed appliances.

1. Patient cooperation is required, even though the appliance is a fixture. The uncooperative patient will not maintain an adequate standard of oral hygiene, will not wear intra-oral elastics or headgear as directed and may intentionally or carelessly damage his or her appliances. Thus fixed appliance treatment is not appropriate for the uncooperative child who will not wear removable appliances. Indeed, in general, a similarly high level of cooperation is required whatever type of orthodontic appliance is selected.
2. The rate of tooth movement is limited by the biological response of the supporting tissues. This is the same, regardless of the type of appliance used.
3. Treatment effects are limited to the teeth and alveolar structures. Whilst it is

possible by controlled tooth movement with fixed appliances to obtain good occlusion even where the skeletal relationship is unfavourable, the improvement in the patient's facial appearance may not match the improvement in occlusion. Where the skeletal pattern is very adverse, it is not possible to obtain a good occlusion, even with fixed appliances. In such situations surgery would be required to correct both the skeletal discrepancy and improve the facial profile.

4. Stability of treatment with fixed appliances depends on exactly the same factors as with removable appliances: the position of balance depends on the harmonious interaction between skeletal relationship, soft tissue pattern and interdental forces. Having stated this, multiple tooth movement is possible with a fixed appliance and therefore careful consideration should be given to the retention phase. In particular, teeth with large rotations are prone to relapse: such corrections should be made early and retained for longer.

Fixed appliance techniques

Multiband techniques

A variety of techniques are available in which attachments are fitted to most or all of the teeth. Archwires are designed so that controlled tooth movement in any plane of space is possible. The most widely known fixed appliance systems are based on the Edgewise and the Begg techniques.

Edgewise technique
This technique is based on a method for moving teeth first described by Edward Angle, the father of modern orthodontics (see Angle, 1928). Attachments with rectangular slots are used (Figure 17.2). Light, small-diameter, round wires may be fitted for initial alignment, but for controlled tooth movement in all planes of space, rectangular archwires, which more closely fit the corresponding slot in the bracket, are used.

Begg technique
In contrast with the Edgewise technique, the attachments have simple vertical slots, which allow free tipping of the teeth (Figure 17.3). Round archwires are used, and controlled root movement in any direction is obtained by the use of auxiliary springs (Begg and Kesling, 1977).

Treatment stages

Whichever technique is selected, treatment may be divided into four main phases.

1. **Alignment phase**. During this initial phase, crowding and rotations are rapidly dealt with to allow the placement of more rigid working archwires. Very flexible wires with large working ranges are used during this early part of treatment. In the past multiple loops might have been bent into a steel wire to allow the distraction of the archwire into the brackets on malpositioned teeth; it is more common in current practice to use thin twisted (braided/

multiflex) steel or preformed superelastic nickel-titanium alloy wires, both of which are very efficient at gaining initial tooth alignment with reduced chairside time.

2. **Working phase**. During this middle period of treatment, horizontal and vertical dento-alveolar corrections are made. Thus the overbite and overjet are reduced. During this phase a more rigid archwire is employed along which the teeth (via the brackets) are generally moved. All spaces are eliminated.

3. **Finishing phase**. Larger archwires more closely fitting the bracket slot are placed. Tooth position is carefully detailed to achieve the best aesthetic and functional result. Where the final archwire is left in place passively for the last 2–3 months this serves as a very effective start to the retention phase.

4. **Retention phase**. The fixed appliance is removed and usually retainers are fitted. These, in contemporary practice, are most usually upper and lower removable appliances designed to fit tightly around the incisors and hold any corrected rotations. The retainers are worn full time for 4–6 months, then at night time only for 4–6 months. Since they are removable they can then be gradually withdrawn to test for tooth stability. There is no absolute rule with regard to a retention regime, every case being treated on its merits. On occasion fixed retainers may be appropriate. These are most commonly employed in the region of the lower incisors, where they might be bonded directly to the lingual surfaces of the lower permanent canines (see Chapter 24).

Fixed-removable appliances

Sometimes it is useful to be able to use fixed attachments in association with a removable appliance. As an example, where the retention of a removable is liable to be poor and it is desirable to use extra-oral traction, bands may be cemented direct to upper molars to carry a facebow (Figure 17.4). This can be used alone to retract the upper molars, or to reinforce anchorage in conjunction with a removable appliance. In that case modified clasps to fit over the tubes on

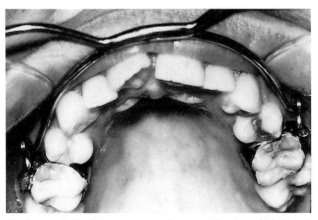

Figure 17.4 Bands cemented to first permanent molars carry tubes into which the ends of the facebow can be fitted. This, together with the headgear, is worn at nights or as prescribed. Some form of safety headgear should always be used (see text and Figure 17.6)

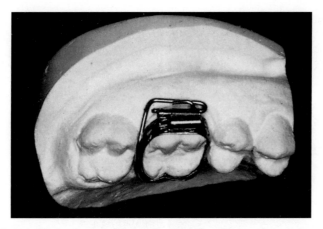

Figure 17.5 A modified molar clasp for an upper removable appliance to be worn in conjunction with the bands on the molars

the molar bands are used on the appliance (Figure 17.5). In either situation, it is wise to incorporate safety mechanisms to reduce the risks of recoil and resultant injuries, which may affect the face, or, in more serious circumstances, the eyes. Such injuries are often due to an incorrect headgear removal procedure, horse-play by the patient or detachment of facebows during sleep. A number of safety mechanisms are available (Figure 17.6); however, they do not reduce the need for careful instructions on fitting, and any patient experiencing detachment of their headgear should return to the clinician as soon as possible. The 'gold standard' are headgears that 'lock' into the fixed appliance.

Where one or perhaps two incisors are rotated, a whip and bonded attachment may be effective when used in conjunction with a labial bow from a removable appliance (Figure 17.7), although a local fixed appliance generally gives better control. By similar means a favourably inclined canine may be drawn across the occlusion from a palatal position (see Figure 17.8a). In both of these examples directly bonded attachments are useful, being connected to the tooth to be moved by the conventional acid/etch technique.

An upper removable appliance may also be used in the early stages of a standard fixed appliance treatment, an anterior bite plane assisting bite opening or clearing the occlusion to allow early lower incisor bracket placement. Gently activated springs mesial to molars may assist the distal movement of these teeth by extra-oral traction (Figure 17.8b).

Segmental fixed appliances

These constitute locally applied fixed appliances generally used in isolation in a buccal or labial segment of the dental arch to improve the tooth alignment. They often form part of an adjunctive treatment (see Chapter 21).

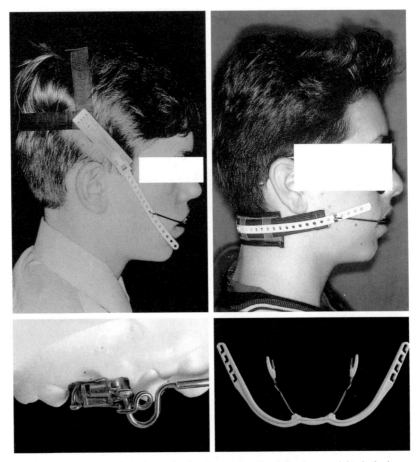

Figure 17.6 Various methods for improving headgear safety. Top left to bottom right clockwise: snap-release; anti-recoil strap; locking catch between inner bow and molar buccal tube; plastic covering all wire ends. (This figure kindly provided by Mr R. Samuels)

Preadjusted fixed appliances

Edgewise

In recent years preadjusted (prescription) versions of the Edgewise appliance have become popular. In such systems, instead of having a simple slot cut in the Edgewise bracket and making adjustments to the tooth position by placing bends or twists in the archwire, each individual tooth correction is built into each bracket slot and/or base. An individual bracket is available for each tooth and carries the average correction for angulation and inclination (torque). Varying the thickness of the bracket base allows the 'in/out' relationship of each tooth to the arch form to be considered. As an example, the average tendency of an upper lateral incisor to be more palatal than the neighbouring central incisor is reflected in a thicker bracket base for the lateral. This detail, which is built into

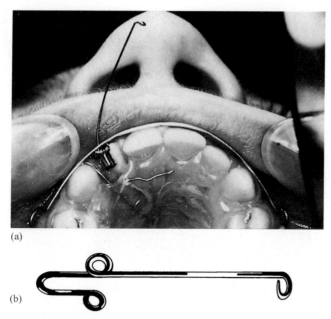

(a)

(b)

Figure 17.7 (a) A whip on the upper lateral incisor with a directly bonded Edgewise bracket. (b) The design of the whip, which is made from 0.5 mm wire. It clips over the wings of the bracket and is held in place by a ligature twisted through the loops in the wire. The free end of the whip clips over the labial bow and a rotational couple is applied to the tooth. The patient can take out the removable appliance for cleaning

every individual bracket, means that flat archwires, of a set curve (preformed in the factory), may be fitted with the minimum of adjustment straight from the packet. In particular, such systems facilitate the use of superelastic (nickel-titanium-based) alloys which have a 'shape memory' and improved flexibility. This generation of archwires place a constant (more physiological) load on a tooth not related to the deflection in order to tie that tooth to the wire.

The advantage of such systems lies in the saving in clinical time and the improved consistency of a good finished result. The disadvantages include cost, the increased stock required and the need for the clinician to recognize the occasional cases where a set prescription in the bracket or archwire is inappropriate.

It is important in any type of fixed appliance mechanism to correctly position the bracket on the crown of the tooth; this is an especially important factor when the main prescription for tooth movement is built into the bracket.

Popular types of Edgewise preadjusted appliances include the systems described by Andrews (1979) or alternatively Roth. These two systems only differ in the prescription (the amount of tip and torque) built into the bracket and base. A case treated by the Roth prescription appliance is shown in Figure 17.9.

Another Edgewise approach is to treat the case in the early stages by sectional arches and then, when the main corrections have been achieved, fit full arches in

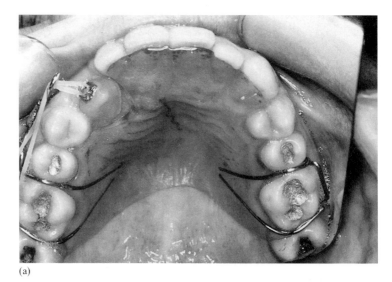

(a)

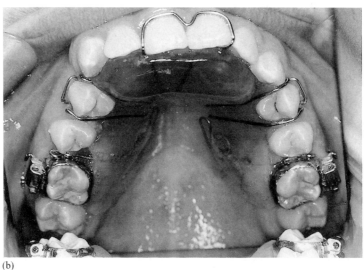

(b)

Figure 17.8 (a) A removable/fixed appliance for moving a canine where the crown is palatal but the root apex is favourably positioned. (b) A removable appliance to support distal movement of upper molars with extra-oral traction. Springs should be only lightly activated. (Case kindly provided by Mr J. Buckley)

a similar manner to conventional Edgewise to finish. An example of such a system is the Bioprogressive technique, as first described by Ricketts (1969). Its advantage lies in minimizing the effects of friction whilst allowing a careful balance of anchorage to be maintained. Its disadvantage lies in the difficulty in controlling tooth movements especially during the early stages of treatment. Figure 17.10 shows a case treated by this technique. A fuller description of the technique is available elsewhere (see Jones *et al.*, 1992).

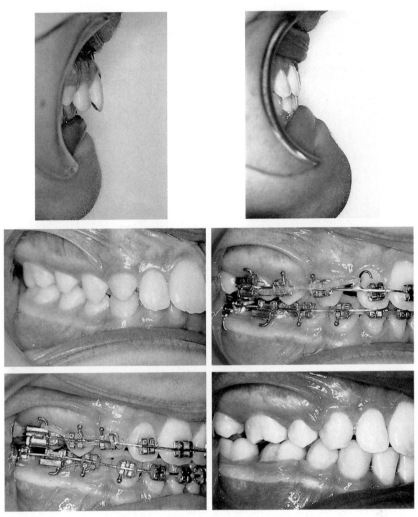

Figure 17.9 A case treated by means of the Roth prescription 'Straight-Wire Appliance' – A preadjusted Edgewise appliance employing full arch mechanics. Middle left to lower right (clockwise) shows sequence of mechanics for a moderate Class II Division 1 case. Note overjet reduction by means of sliding mechanics along the archwire, the force being provided by intramaxillary elastic traction whilst the anchor molars are held in position by headgear. The upper views show start to finish overjet. (Records of the case kindly provided by Dr J. Knox)

Begg

A preadjusted version of the Begg appliance is also available, called Tip-Edge. In this system the early stages of treatment follow conventional lines (Figure 17.3); however, the bracket includes a preadjusted element similar to the Edge-wise bracket which facilitates the fitting of a rectangular finishing wire at the end of treatment. The progress of treatment is shown for a typical Class II Division 1 Tip-Edge case in Figure 17.11.

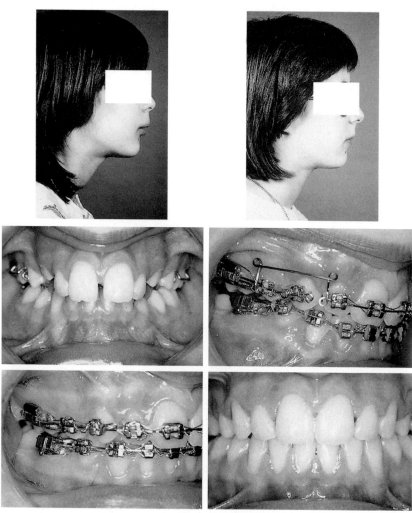

Figure 17.10 A case treated by means of the Bioprogressive technique – a version of a preadjusted Edgewise appliance employing sectional mechanics. Middle left to lower right (clockwise) shows the sequence of mechanics. Initially a space maintainer has been fitted to both hold space following extraction and start bite opening. After the upper canines have erupted they have been retracted using a sectional archwire (see also Figure 21.3). Next the overjet has been reduced using another section termed a 'utility'. Finally, full archwires have been fitted to respond to the prescription in the bracket and facilitate individual tooth positioning. The upper views show the before and after facial profile. (Records of the case kindly provided by Ms H. Taylor)

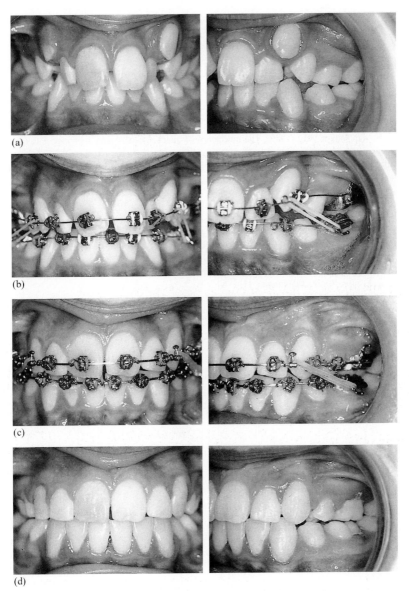

(a)

(b)

(c)

(d)

Figure 17.11 Treatment with the prescription 'Tip-Edge' appliance. This is derived from the original Begg appliance. A typical treatment of a Class II Division 1 malocclusion is shown. (a) Original malocclusion. (b) Completion of alignment phase – addition of Class II elastics is 'driving' the overjet reduction. (c) 'Detailing phase' – rectangular archwire and auxiliary springs in place. (d) The post-treatment result on day of appliance removal (debond)

Further reading

Andrews, F. (1979). The straight wire appliance. *British Journal of Orthodontics*, **6**, 125–43.

Angle, E. (1928). The latest and best in orthodontic mechanisms. *Dental Cosmos*, **70**, 1143–58.

Begg, P.R. and Kesling, P.C. (1977). *Begg Orthodontic Theory and Technique*, 3rd edn. Philadelphia: W.B. Saunders.

Bowden, D.E.J. (1978). Theoretical considerations of headgear. Parts 1 & 2. *British Journal of Orthodontics*, **5**, 145–52, 173–81.

Evans, T.J.W., Jones, M.L. and Newcombe, R.G. (1997). A clinical comparison and performance perspective of three aligning archwires. *American Journal of Orthodontics and Dentofacial Orthopedics*, **114**, 32–9.

Jones, M.L., Nicholson, P.T., Oliver, R.G. and Robertson, N.R.E. (1992). The place of the Bioprogressive technique in postgraduate teaching. *British Journal of Orthodontics*, **19**, 1–13.

Jones, S. and Waters, N.E. (1989). The mechanics of quadhelix expansion appliance. Parts 1 & 2. *European Journal of Orthodontics*, **11**, 169–78, 195–9.

Kesling, P.C. (1989). Dynamics of the tip-edge bracket. *American Journal of Orthodontics and Dentofacial Orthopaedics*, **96**, 16–25.

Ricketts, R.M. (1969). Bioprogressive therapy as an answer to orthodontic needs. Part 1. *American Journal of Orthodontics*, **70**, 241–68.

Roth, R. (1994). Treatment mechanics for the straight wire appliance. In *Orthodontics: Current Principles and Practice*, 2nd edn. (T.M. Graber and R.L. Vanarsdall, eds) St Louis: Mosby.

Samuels, R.H.A. and Jones, M.L. (1994). Orthodontic facebow injuries and safety equipment. *European Journal of Orthodontics*, **16**, 385–94.

Tweed, C.H. (1941). The application of the principles of the edgewise arch in the treatment of malocclusions. *Angle Orthodontist*, **11**, 5–67.

Waters, N.E., Houston, W.J.B. and Stephens, C.D. (1981). The characterisation of archwires for the initial alignment of irregular teeth. *American Journal of Orthodontics*, **66**, 487–97.

Chapter 18

Treatment with functional appliances

Functional appliances utilize the forces of the orofacial musculature to move teeth. The fact that they depend on muscle forces in no way implies a special mode of action: they produce their effects as a result of tooth movement brought about by the tissue changes described in Chapter 15. The major effect of functional appliances is on the position of the teeth and alveolar processes, in other words the correction of the malocclusion is largely by dento-alveolar camouflage. There is still much debate about the possibility of orthopaedic change, with some evidence that in favourable cases mandibular condylar growth may be modified or redirected.

Many functional appliances have been described but only the more important examples from each group will be mentioned in this text. For a more detailed account of their use and construction see Adams and Kerr (1990), Isaacson *et al.* (1990) or Orton (1990).

The Andresen appliance

This appliance (Figure 18.1a) was developed from the monobloc of Robin (1902). It consists of upper and lower appliances sealed together with the mandibular arch postured, so that the forces of the muscles of mastication can be transmitted between the dental arches. This produces an intermaxillary type of force which acts to correct the Class II type of antero-posterior arch discrepancy.

Although a variety of malocclusions may be treated by the expert, the general use of the Andresen appliance is confined to carefully selected Class II Division 1 cases with the following classically described features:

1. The arches must be uncrowded and in regular alignment. It is advantageous if the upper incisors are spaced. The upper molars must not be inclined distally.
2. The lower arch should not normally be more than a half cusp width distal to the upper.
3. The skeletal pattern should be ideally Class I or mild Class II.
4. There must be no habit posture of the mandible.
5. Ideally the patient should not have entered their prepubertal growth spurt.

For success, the working bite and laboratory procedures must be carried out carefully. The working bite is taken with the mandible symmetrically postured

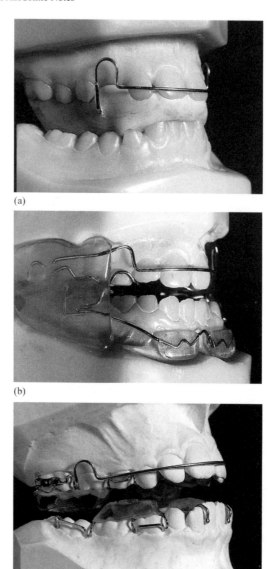

(a)

(b)

(c)

Figure 18.1 (a) An Andresen appliance (the bite has been postured forwards in this Class II Division 1 case – in this instance it is more open than classically described). (b) A Frankel appliance (the bite has been postured forwards into the appliance to correct the Class II Division 1 malocclusion). (c) Clark's twin-block appliance (in this adaptation of the appliance headgear tubes are also included; the models have been opened for the purposes of illustration in this Class II Division 1 case – note the angled posterior bite-blocks which serve to posture the mandible forwards on closure)

forwards to obtain a Class I buccal segment relationship and opened about 2 mm beyond the freeway space. This means that when the appliance is fitted the mandible is held forwards and the muscles acting on it (in particular the posterior fibres of temporalis) tend to retract it to its normal position. As a result forces are generated which tend to move the upper teeth distally and the lower teeth mesially. This is an example of intermaxillary traction. In order to facilitate tooth movement and allow overbite reduction, channels are trimmed over the occlusal surfaces of the molars and premolars. These channels are directed backwards in the upper arch and forwards in the lower. As a result, the appliance contacts the upper posterior teeth only on their mesiopalatal aspects and the lowers only on their distolingual aspects. This guides their direction of eruption to encourage correction of the occlusion. It is important that, in the construction of the appliance, the acrylic should be carried over the lower incisor tips. The capping acts as a bite plane to permit overbite reduction and is meant to prevent the lower incisors from tipping forwards. However, a major problem with the Andresen appliance is that the lower incisors may be moved labially out of muscle balance and therefore could relapse when treatment is completed.

The patient is instructed to wear the appliance at night and for as many hours as possible each day. With careful case selection good results may be obtained, but the clinician needs to make a careful assessment of the facial profile before prescribing a functional appliance: where a true maxillary protrusion is present, such cases may more readily be treated by using a more conventional appliance. For example, the mild uncrowded Class II Division I malocclusion may be treated by using extra-oral traction to retract the upper buccal segments, followed by overjet reduction, without any risk of disturbing the balance of the lower arch.

The Harvold appliance

This appliance, which is also known as the Harvold activator (Harvold and Vargevick, 1971), belongs to a group of essentially tooth-borne appliances which all derive from the original design of Andresen. It differs in that it holds the teeth further apart thus exhibiting a greater potential for both bite opening and intermaxillary traction. It is also trimmed differently in that the appliance's lingual flange is constructed to be well clear of the teeth of the lower buccal segments: this allows the teeth of the lower buccal segments to erupt upwards and forwards to assist both the overbite and the horizontal molar correction.

The very large amount of vertical opening is intended to take advantage of a theoretical muscular and soft tissue recoil to correct the Class II arch relationship. However, such a degree of opening can also make the appliance uncomfortable to wear.

The Frankel appliance

This is a variety of functional appliance (Figure 18.1b) which differs from the Andresen appliance in that its action primarily depends on acrylic shields which are designed to hold the lips and cheeks away from the teeth, so disturbing the muscle balance and producing tooth movement. This appliance has been described as being soft-tissue-borne rather than tooth-borne, the latter being the case with most other appliances in the family of functionals. In Class II cases, the appliance is designed to hold the mandible in a forward position.

The appliance is described by Frankel (1980) as a 'function regulator' (FR) and, as its name implies, he believes that it permanently modifies the position and activities of the orofacial muscles and promotes growth at the mandibular condyle. At present there is no objective evidence to support these views. Treatment with the Frankel appliance is usually begun in the early mixed dentition. The appliance is worn part time until the patient is accustomed to it, then full time. Although the appropriately designed Frankel appliance can theoretically be used to treat any arch malrelationship, it is used most commonly in Class II Division 1 malocclusions. Crowding in Class II cases is not a contra-indication for its use since some arch expansion is produced, but clearly the result will not be stable unless the teeth are in a position of muscle balance at the end of treatment.

Clark's Twin-Block appliance

This tooth-borne functional appliance has become very popular in recent years for the treatment of moderate to severe Class II Division 1 type malocclusions. It differs from the Andresen in that the upper and lower components of the appliance are not sealed together, being free to move apart when the patient opens their mouth. On closure (Figure 18.1c), angled posterior bite blocks on the upper and lower plates guide the occlusion into a postured position, similar to that obtained with other functionals. The principal advantage of the twin block is that it is better tolerated than most functionals and is therefore worn for longer to achieve a more rapid correction of the antero-posterior arch discrepancy. As with other functional appliances, it is usually unwise to attempt a full horizontal occlusal correction in one go. Accordingly, the mandibular arch should not be initially postured forwards by much more than 7 mm, otherwise the appliance may prove uncomfortable and will not be worn. Clark's appliance may be activated quite easily during treatment by adding acrylic to the blocks (see Clark, 1988).

In both Clark and Frankel appliances the likely effect on the facial profile of a successful treatment may be rehearsed by asking the patient to posture the mandible forwards to a Class I incisor relationship.

Activators for use with fixed appliances

There are now available a range of 'cut-down' activators based on the earlier design described above. However, these appliances are less bulky, easier to wear and as a result may be worn simultaneously with a twin arch fixed appliance. This obviously has major advantages in being able to correct the underlying Class II dental arch discrepancy whilst dealing with arch alignment of teeth. These appliances were first described by Orton and are discussed in more detail in his excellent text on functional appliances (see Orton, 1990).

Adjunctive appliances to support functionals

There are a variety of appliances that may be used to facilitate, support or retain a functional treatment. The use of a fixed appliance either during or after treatment with a functional has been mentioned already. However, upper arch retained removable appliances also have a role:

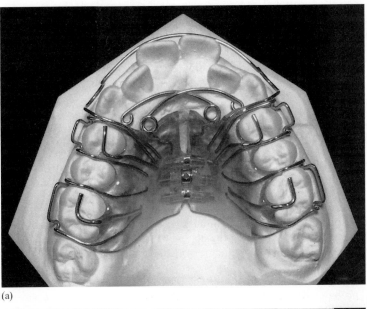

(a)

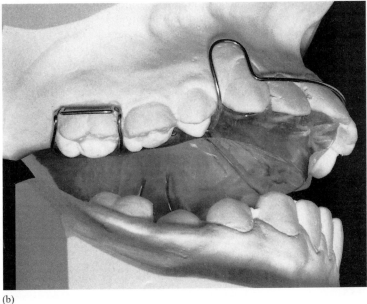

(b)

Figure 18.2 (a) An '*ELSAA*' appliance (see text). Such types of removable appliance are used to prepare the maxillary dental arch to receive the definitive functional appliance. This one expands the upper arch whilst aligning the labial segment. (b) An example of a second-stage appliance for use after the correction of a Class II Division 1 malocclusion with a functional. The angled upper anterior bite-plane helps to retain the overjet correction whilst allowing the buccal segments to settle into their final horizontal and vertical relationship

- They may be used to expand the maxillary arch and align the labial segment prior to the functional phase of treatment. An example of this is the ELSAA (**E**xpansion & **L**abial **S**egment **A**lignment **A**ppliances) (Figure 18.2a).
- They may be used as post-functional retainers. This can be achieved through the construction of a second-stage appliance which has an angled anterior bite plane to support the overjet reduction whilst allowing the buccal segments the freedom to drift into an improved vertical and horizontal position (Figure 18.2b).

Conclusions

A very large number of functional appliances have been described in the literature, unfortunately there have been very few scientifically valid studies to investigate how they achieve correction of the malocclusion. However, it would appear that much of the change in dental arch relationship is achieved by a combination of dento-alveolar camouflage and favourable growth of the jaws. For the best chance of success the appliance must be worn for lengthy periods and the treatment timed to coincide with the individual's growth spurt. Since both of these factors are, to a large extent, outside the control of the clinician it is wise to review progress carefully. If little change is seen after six months it would probably be sensible to consider other possible treatment options.

At their most effective, functional appliances are very valuable in that they provide a possible treatment in the mixed dentition for significant horizontal dental arch discrepancies. Although they may be employed in other types of malocclusion they appear to be most useful in Class II Division 1 types. Once the overjet is corrected a fixed appliance can be fitted subsequently to allow detail tooth alignment.

Further reading

Adams, C.P. and Kerr, W.J.S. (1990). *The Design and Use of Removable Orthodontic Appliances*, 6th edn. Oxford: Butterworth-Heinemann.

Clark, W.J. (1988). The twin block technique. *American Journal of Orthodontics*, **93**, 1–18.

Clark, W.J. (1995). *Twin Block Functional Therapy, Applications in Dentofacial Orthopaedics*. London: Times-Mirror.

Frankel, R. (1980). A functional approach to orofacial orthopaedics. *British Journal of Orthodontics*, **7**, 41–5.

Harvold, E.P. and Vargevick, K. (1971). Morphogenetic response to activator treatment. *American Journal of Orthodontics*, **60**, 478–90.

Isaacson, K.G., Reed, R.T. and Stephens, C.D. (1990). *Functional Orthodontic Appliances*. Oxford: Blackwell Scientific Publications.

Orton, H.S. (1990). *Functional Appliances in Orthodontic Treatment*. London: Quintessence Publishing.

Chapter 19

Radiology in orthodontics

The importance and value of radiographs in diagnosis and treatment planning is well documented. However, a radiograph should never be taken unless it offers a 'benefit' to the patient that outweighs the 'risk' of the radiation exposure. *Therefore, the orthodontic clinician should be able to justify the taking of each radiograph as being to the advantage of each individual patient.* Taking a radiograph cannot be justified on medicolegal grounds alone. Interpretation should be made only from good quality radiographs in terms both of technique and processing.

This chapter gives a brief account of the main projections used in orthodontics, the main clinical indications for radiography, and some recommendations to assist the clinician in matching the appropriate view with the information required. Bearing in mind the biological effects and risks of X-rays, the practitioner has ethical and legal obligations to minimize the radiation dose to patients, practitioner, staff and public.

Radiation dose

The **absorbed dose** measures the amount of energy imparted by radiation to a unit mass of tissue. It is expressed in a unit of measurement termed the **gray** (symbol: Gy). Since equal absorbed doses from various radiations (e.g. X-rays, alpha particles) do not necessarily have equal biological effects, another quantity is needed. This is the **dose equivalent**, which is expressed in a unit of measurement called the **sievert** (symbol: Sv). Dose equivalent is equal to the absorbed dose multiplied by a factor that takes account of the way a particular radiation distributes energy within tissue, thus influencing its effectiveness in causing harm. The risk of fatal malignancy or hereditary damage per sievert is not the same for all tissue types. For example, it is lower for the thyroid than for the testes or ovaries. For this reason, the dose equivalent in each of the major organs and tissues of the body is subject to a weighting factor related to the individual risk to that organ. The sum of these corrected measurements is termed the **effective dose equivalent** and it is recorded in sieverts.

The word 'dose' is applied loosely to the **effective dose equivalent**, and the units millisievert (mSv) and, more usually, microsievert (μSv) are used. The average radiation dose from different radiological examinations, together with the estimated risk and equivalent period of natural background radiation, is

Table 19.1 Mean effective dose equivalents from different radiological examinations – estimated risk per million of a fatal cancer†

X-ray examination	Effective dose (μSv)	Estimated risk per million of a fatal cancer	Equivalent period of natural background radiation*
Intra-oral (periapical, bitewing, upper standard occlusal)	2–10	0.06–0.7	1 day
Oblique lateral (bimolar)	2–8	0.06–0.7	1 day
Dental panoramic	7–26	0.21–1.9	1–6 days
Lateral cephalometric	3	0.06–0.1	2.5 days
Skull	100	6.0	17 days
Chest	20–40	0.2	3–7 days
Barium meal	5000	265	2.1 years

*There are inconsistencies in the literature because of differences in method of calculation.
†Estimate of average dose per year for each inhabitant of the UK is 2200 μSv.

given in Table 19.1. Effective dose is calculated for any X-ray technique by measuring the energy absorption in a number of 'key' organs in the body, so that the final figure is a representation of 'whole body' detriment.

No dose of radiation can be considered as safe, no matter how small. However, the small risks involved in dental radiography should be kept in perspective.

Paediatric radiography

Radiation risk is age-dependent, being the highest for the young and the lowest for the elderly. The risk of cancer is tripled for the age group 0–10 years, and doubled for those aged 10–20 years (see ICRP, 1990).

The majority of orthodontic patients are children. Since they are both growing and developing, their tissues are generally at higher risk from radiation. Therefore, it is important that radiation protection procedures are rigidly enforced.

Generally, children require smaller radiation doses than adults since their tissues are reduced both in thickness and density. As a consequence, it is often possible to employ a reduced exposure time or a lower milliamperage. Since children have a tendency to move when radiographs are being taken, it is best to decrease the exposure time rather than the milliamperage. This prevents blurring and produces a more consistently sharp image.

Measures and factors modifying effective dose

In addition to the use of well-maintained and monitored X-ray equipment and a high standard of radiographic technique, the operator must never stand in the direct line of the main beam. It is best to stand behind a lead barrier or no closer than 1.5 metres (6 ft) to the unit during an exposure, and preferably at right-angles to the beam. The following general measures should also be followed.

Selection criteria

Prescription of radiographs should be based on the history and clinical findings, and they must only be undertaken when the investigation is likely to affect the management of the patient in terms of diagnosis and treatment. Decisions should be based on the information required. Important factors are:

- the likely abnormality being investigated and its extent
- whether a general or detailed view is necessary
- whether the patient is new to the clinic or has been recalled
- whether special radiological or scanning techniques are indicated.

The frequency with which films are taken will depend upon the availability and timing of previous radiographs, together with any monitoring regimen that is being pursued. However, it is important that radiography is not seen as a 'routine' procedure that automatically accompanies a periodic recall examination. Radiographic screening of children for malocclusion has not been shown to be of benefit to the community at large and, in general, is not recommended.

Quality assurance programme

The purpose of a quality assurance programme is to produce radiographs that are of high quality with maximum diagnostic information, while using the least amount of radiation. They should also be produced at minimum financial cost. This programme includes processing and darkroom quality control.

The following factors modify effective dose:

- method of X-ray generation (pulsating or constant potential)
- exposure factors (kilo voltage, milliampere-seconds – mAs)
- filtration (to absorb 'soft' low-energy radiation from the beam)
- collimation (to restrict the volume of the beam to the area of interest)
- cone length (focus to skin distance – fsd)
- image receptor (film speed, film/screen speed, or digital system): e.g. rare-earth intensifying screens significantly reduce radiation without affecting the diagnostic yield
- lead apron and thyroid collar.

General orthodontic indications for dental radiographs

Intra- and extra-oral views

The main function of **lateral cephalometric skull** films is to produce a record of the developing face and dentition (see Figure 4.2). The need, use and analysis of such films have been discussed previously in Chapter 4. **Postero-anterior (PA) skull** views may be of use in patients presenting with facial asymmetry and may occasionally be helpful in the assessment of certain jaw or dental anomalies.

For general assessment and when dental panoramic tomography is not available, right and left lateral oblique or bimolar projections (Figure 19.1) may be taken, together with upper and lower standard (central oblique) occlusals.

The bimolar is an oblique lateral projection designed to show premolars and molars in both jaws on the same radiograph. By careful application of a lead

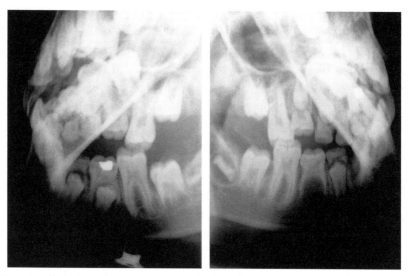

Figure 19.1 Bimolar or lateral oblique radiographs. Note the congenital absence of the maxillary second premolar on the patient's right side (left radiograph) and congenital absence of the mandibular second premolar on the patient's left side (right radiograph). The artefact on the left radiograph below the border of the mandible is a metal stud-fastener on the patient's jacket

screen to cover half of the cassette at each exposure, it is possible to fit both sides of the jaws on one film.

The **upper standard occlusal** is usually taken together with a **dental panoramic tomogram** particularly where there are reasonable grounds for suspecting that pathology exists, or when searching for a supernumerary tooth or an odontome. This occlusal view provides additional information in 20% of instances to contemporary panoramic radiography. A small mesiodens can sometimes be missed on panoramic projections if it lies outside the focal trough or is resorbing.

The vertex occlusal film is taken with the X-ray beam aimed down the root of the upper incisors. It gives a plan view of the upper arch and has often been used in the past to localize an unerupted upper canine. However, this projection is not recommended for regular use in contemporary practice, as it gives an unacceptable level of radiation dose for usually poor contrast and detail. On the rare occasions that it proves necessary to employ this view, a dental X-ray set with a capability in excess of 65 kV should be employed, together with an intra-oral cassette containing intensifying screens. A lead apron should protect the gonads. Whenever intra-oral periapical radiography is employed, a paralleling technique, with film-holder and beam-aiming device is recommended.

The panoramic or bimolar projections may need to be supplemented by appropriate periapical films where additional fine detail might be necessary, as in suspicion of root resorption, dilaceration or other similar dental malformations.

Dental panoramic tomograph (DPT)

This film is useful when a comprehensive dental examination, including dental development, anomalies and pathology of the jaws, is desirable (see Figure 8.6).

The temporomandibular joints and maxillary sinuses are also depicted. This projection is relatively easy to perform and has the added value of a reduction of radiation when compared with a series of full-mouth intra-oral films. This latter approach would be rarely indicated in the orthodontic clinic.

It is important to appreciate that the DPT differs from conventional radiographs by being a sectional radiograph, and only the structures within the section (focal trough or zone of sharpness) will be in focus in the final image. The other structures on both sides of the section will be blurred and degrade the picture.

The principles of panoramic imaging are described in specialized textbooks (see Whaites, 1996). The discussion here will be confined only to important points, which should be understood as they influence both image quality and interpretation.

Since the DPT has a predetermined focal trough corresponding to the average shape of the dental arch, the distortion and unsharpness of the image increases as the dental arch diverges from the norm. The focal trough narrows anteriorly, which means that often even a quite small positioning error of the incisor teeth could greatly distort the local image. Magnification in panoramic radiography is complex because the ratio of the focus–object to the object–film distance is not everywhere identical. Magnification also varies across the film and from patient to patient. In practical terms this means that the size of teeth may be over- or underestimated, and the inclination/angulation of teeth cannot be accurately perceived.

Common artefacts might include ghost images of the hard palate and nasal structures (usually overlapping the maxillary sinus of the opposite side), the mandibular ramus of the other side and cervical vertebrae. Ghost images are the result of the projection of structures that are positioned between the X-ray source and the centre of rotation. They are seen on the opposite side of the film enlarged, distorted and at a higher level from the real shadows.

In order to obtain a diagnostic-quality panoramic image, free of both artefacts and positioning errors, the patient must be prepared (i.e. hair slides, spectacles, nose and/or earrings and studs, and intra-oral appliances should all be removed). The patient should then be positioned in the machine with the mid-sagittal plane perpendicular to the floor, and the Frankfort plane roughly parallel to the floor. The anterior teeth should be centred in the focal trough and the neck should be extended. A common pitfall is the positioning error when the chin is raised too high and as a consequence the roots of the maxillary anterior teeth are 'cut off', mimicking root resorption.

Further notes on panoramic radiography

1. Where there is an extreme discrepancy in the facial skeleton (Class II or III) the anterior teeth relationships may make it impossible to obtain a clear image of the maxillary and mandibular anterior segments simultaneously. In patients with an Angle's Class II Division 1 malocclusion, it might be necessary to lift the face slightly during positioning. In Class II Division 2, it may be advisable for the patient to occlude on a cotton roll during exposure to avoid a vertical overlap of the teeth.

2. In the buccal regions, the maxillary teeth show much more overlap than those in the mandible. The image of the hard palate usually overlaps the unerupted teeth or the developing roots.

3. Evaluation of space. In the developing dentition, accurate space measurement is seriously limited. In general, angular measurements are more reliable in the buccal areas. Usually linear dimensions in the vertical direction are enlarged by a more constant factor, whereas in the horizontal direction this effect is more variable, increasing from the mesial part of the film back to the distal.
4. The DPT is of limited use in the evaluation of patients with jaw and other dental asymmetries.
5. A new generation of panoramic radiographic machines has arrived with the development of the 'Scanora R'. This apparatus incorporates zonography software, which permits tomography of the temporomandibular joint or cross-section of the jaw. A current drawback to such equipment is the high cost, and its value in the orthodontic context still awaits assessment. Among other developments is the increased availability of digital imaging, which may become more widely used in the near future. The eventual intention is to replace film-based technology with computer-based devices that may record and then store the image in a digital form.

Localization of unerupted or misplaced teeth

The basis for the localization technique is a change in positional reference (object and the reference object) that results from altering the central ray projection. The relative object–film distance may provide clues: objects closer to a film appear sharper and of actual size; objects distant to the film appear more blurred and enlarged.

One method of location is by the application of two different projections (that are at right-angles to each other). Another technique, frequently employed in orthodontics, is the parallax method, where one standard projection is taken and then the tube is shifted either horizontally or vertically with a resultant change in the central ray projection. As an example, a standard (central oblique) occlusal film may be used together with an appropriate peri-apical to locate an unerupted maxillary canine (Figure 19.2). On each film the image of the root of the lateral incisor and the crown of the canine will be visible. The image, which moves in the same direction as the X-ray tube, is the palatally or lingually placed object. Likewise, the object, which moves in the opposite direction to the movement of the tube, is buccal or labial.

Panoramic radiographs also may assist in tooth location. In the plane of the film, objects that lie in front of the image layer (focal trough) are blurred and reduced in size, whereas those that are behind the image layer appear out of focus and enlarged.

Phases of orthodontic radiography

Orthodontic radiographic examinations can be considered in four phases:

1. **Pretreatment phase**. General radiographic assessment as an aid to diagnosis and treatment planning is particularly helpful where extractions and/or apical movements are being considered, and also when local pathology needs to be

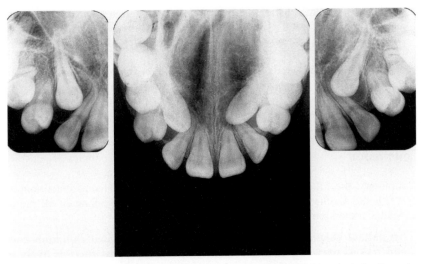

Figure 19.2 Anterior maxillary root length occlusal radiograph (centre) with periapical radiographs of the right and left maxillary canine regions. Relative to the root of the lateral incisor, on both sides the shadow of the unerupted canine has moved in the same direction as the movement of the X-ray tube. This indicates that the unerupted maxillary canines are palatally placed

excluded. A dental panoramic tomograph or alternatively left/right oblique lateral (bimolar) views, together with the appropriate occlusal radiographs, are often indicated to provide an initial scan of the teeth and jaws in a new patient. True cephalometric lateral skull views are taken to aid orthodontic diagnosis and treatment planning, especially in cases of suspected skeletal discrepancy. Such films may provide a baseline for the monitoring of treatment, provided that they have been properly analysed (see Chapter 4) by tracing or computer digitization. It should be emphasized that there is no evidence that a single cephalometric view is of use in the prediction of facial growth, and a single film should not be taken solely for this purpose.

2. **Monitoring (mid-treatment) phase**. In many cases the more experienced orthodontic clinician requires few monitoring radiographs. However, in more severe cases of malocclusion and/or when two-arch fixed appliance techniques are being used, lateral cephalometric views may be necessary for periodical assessment of treatment progress. Intra-oral radiographs, including standard occlusal views, may also be indicated to assess the progress of unerupted teeth or when root resorption is suspected, evidence of the latter being hypermobility of the teeth or where the root apices are initially blunted, thin or spindly.

3. **End of active treatment phase**. Routine radiographs taken at the end of active treatment do not generally benefit the individual patient. However, there are situations where long-term stability is less certain, due to the treatment itself, to aetiological factors or to the unpredictability of future growth. Such cases may require radiographs to provide a baseline from which to assess further changes. Post-treatment films are of most value to a clinician's learning process, when they are collected to a set regimen,

particularly when constituting part of an accepted research protocol or auditing process. In such situations the taking of films is justified as being of benefit to the population as a whole (see National Radiological Protection Board, 1994).

4. **Post-retention phase**. Radiographic examination during the post-retention phase is usually not necessary for the future management of the patient. However, films may be justified in selected cases where there is a clinical indication or as part of the structured learning process mentioned previously.

Conclusion

In summary, the following statement (Faculty of General Dental Practitioners, 1998) should be the guiding international principle in the taking of all radiographs for orthodontic purposes:

No patient should be expected to receive any additional radiation dose and risk as part of a course of dental treatment unless there is likely to be a benefit in terms of improved management of that patient

Further reading

British Orthodontic Society (1994, 2000). *Orthodontic Radiography Guidelines.* London: BOS.

Faculty of General Dental Practitioners (1998). *Selection Criteria for Dental Radiography.* London: Royal College of Surgeons of England.

ICRP (1990). Recommendations of the International Commission on Radiological Protection 60. *Annals of the ICRP,* **21**, 1–3.

National Radiological Protection Board (1994). *Guidelines on Radiology Standards for Primary Dental Care.* NRPB Vol. 5, No. 3. London: HMSO.

Whaites, E. (1996). *Essentials of Dental Radiography and Radiology,* 2nd edn. London: Churchill Livingstone.

Chapter 20

Dento-alveolar surgery in relation to orthodontics

Introduction

The specialties of oral surgery and orthodontics relate closely to one another in a number of ways. Minor surgical procedures can facilitate and expedite treatment, improve the periodontal condition, reduce relapse, add to post-orthodontic stability and improve dental aesthetics for orthodontic patients. There are also a number of surgical procedures which have been specifically designed with orthodontic treatment in mind.

A team approach, with discussion about the type and timing of surgery, is essential. This should also include discussion about possible alternatives to treatment and any anaesthetic proposed.

General principles

Preoperative assessment

One of the problems of a joint approach is the risk that one party erroneously assumes that the other has performed a particular task. For example, all patients should have a thorough medical history taken and recorded in the patient's file. This would include conditions which might affect wound healing or suscept-ibility to infection, and identification of those who require prophylactic anti-biotic cover. It is also important to obtain information on bleeding disorders, allergies and medications which might complicate any planned procedures.

Initially, the proposed procedure should be fully explained to both the child and the parents. This explanation includes an outline of advantages, disadvan-tages and possible complications so that the patient, parent or guardian may give informed consent. Anxieties should be alleviated as far as possible and plans made for any premedication that may be necessary.

A decision to recommend a particular type of anaesthetic should be made on clinical grounds, local being preferable to general wherever possible. Clinical judgment must also be employed to assess whether children are capable of coping with the stress of a minor oral surgical procedure without being put off dentistry for life. Where there is some doubt, sedation techniques may offer an acceptable alternative mode of treatment.

Operative considerations

The general principles of good surgical technique should be applied to minor oral surgery as much as to any other procedure. Despite the remarkable ability of the mouth to heal well, the risk of infection remains considerable and can be minimized by use of an aseptic technique and appropriate antibiotic prescribing. The use of steroids is seldom indicated for simple minor oral surgical procedures prior to orthodontics.

Surgical incisions should be made cleanly and safely, bearing in mind the proximity of any anatomically important structures. Wherever possible, the design of the flap should be such that it is firmly based on bone, has a wide base and narrows at its apex, is parallel to the muscle insertions where present and can easily be repaired. The flap should be large enough to provide good access and visibility whilst minimizing trauma to the tissues. Incisions around the cervical margin should be relieved vertically by elevating the whole of the interdental papilla, rather than splitting it in half. Care must always be taken with the retraction of the flap during the operative procedure.

When bone removal is necessary, this can be undertaken with surgical burs or sharp chisels. Occasionally bone-nibbling forceps such as Rongeurs can be used. When the patient is anaesthetized, a chisel is more efficient and less traumatic than a bur to expose a tooth crown or root. It may also be used as a hand instrument under local anaesthetic to 'shave' bone and gently expose a site. At the end of the procedure the wound should be irrigated and cleansed with sterile saline to remove any debris. Sharp bone edges should be filed or smoothed with a suitable bur, haemostasis achieved and the wound closed.

When replacing the flap, the margins should be approximated accurately over bone and should not be overlapped. The corners of the flap are sutured first, starting with the mobile corner to the fixed. The sutures must not be too tight and the knots should be away from the incision to prevent irritation. There is good evidence that excessive suturing causes increased swelling so sutures should be placed with enough space to allow for some drainage. This will help to minimize swelling and the likelihood of any haematoma formation. When a flap cannot be replaced over bone for some reason, it may be helpful to use horizontal mattress sutures to ensure the flap edges evert and thus promote healing by primary intention.

Postoperative instructions

The importance of adequate postoperative instructions cannot be emphasized enough. Patients should be informed as to the likely progress of the healing process and given appropriate analgesia. Antibiotics should be prescribed if there is a significant risk of infection, but in preorthodontic minor oral surgery this is rarely the case. Instructing a patient in good oral hygiene techniques and the use of antiseptic mouthwashes, such as chlorhexidine, is usually more than adequate for most patients.

Verbal and written instructions must be provided with details of whom to contact in the event of a postoperative complication (e.g. bleeding). Finally, arrangements should be made for any review either to remove packs/sutures, etc. or to assess the need for, and timing of, future orthodontics.

Common oro-surgical procedures for orthodontics

There are basically three types of oral surgical procedures for orthodontics. These are:

1. Surgery on the soft tissues.
2. Surgery relating to unerupted or misplaced teeth.
3. Surgery on the hard tissues.

Some of the more common procedures are outlined below.

Surgery on the soft tissues

Fraenectomy

Fraenectomies may be carried out on maxillary and mandibular fraena. The presence of a gap (diastema) between the maxillary central incisors may be accompanied by a low attachment of the labial fraenum which, in severe cases, can even merge with the incisive papilla. It has been suggested that if the fraenum is removed, the space may be closed with appliances more easily.

Fraenectomy is an operation designed to remove the entire fraenum and, if necessary, the fibrous tissue lying in the intermaxillary suture between the roots of the central incisor teeth. A fraenectomy may be performed at two main times:

1. In the early transitional dentition, when an extremely large diastema (6–8 mm) is present. This procedure facilitates space closure and may prevent ectopic eruption of the lateral incisors and/or canines. On occasion it may lead to some spontaneous space closure without orthodontic treatment, but this is unpredictable;
2. In the late transitional dentition, following the complete eruption of the lateral incisors together with the canines and where the diastema has failed to close naturally.

A V-shaped radiographic appearance of the interproximal bone between the maxillary central incisors is a useful diagnostic sign that a fibrous fraenum contributing to the diastema is present; it is also an indicator that it may require removal.

The surgical techniques for performing a fraenectomy are described in detail in several specialized textbooks (see Further reading). However, there are several points worth emphasizing. When the fraenum is relatively thin but simply attached too low, a horizontal incision can be made into the midpoint of the fraenum. This creates a rhomboid-shaped wound, the edges of which can be undermined prior to suturing. Since no tissue is actually excised, the results tend to be extremely good with minimal scarring. In cases where the fraenum is thick and fleshy, it should be partially excised using two vertical incisions. When these join palatally on the tip of the incisive papilla, the tissue on the mesial aspect of both central incisors should be left. This is very important for the regeneration of the interdental papilla, and gives an improved aesthetic result. It is also important to clear completely all fibrous tissue from the median suture and, on rare occasions where excessive bone is found in the suture, this should be reduced with a bur.

An enlarged mandibular labial fraenum is comparatively rare compared with the maxillary fraenum but, when present, it may contribute to movement of the marginal gingiva around the lower central incisors when the keratinized tissue has been lost, reduced, detached or where mechanical trauma exists. In these situations a simple fraenectomy is unlikely to be adequate and a free gingival graft should be considered.

The mandibular lingual fraenum, with high attachment to the alveolar ridge between the lower central incisors, may also contribute to a diastema. If necessary it can be divided horizontally near the alveolar ridge and, if the wound is large, sutured vertically. Many cases require no suturing at all. The usual cause of complaint regarding the lingual fraenum is that of a child being tongue-tied. In itself this is not an indication to undertake surgery, particularly in the very young.

In older children lingual fraenectomy should only be considered if:

- the child cannot place his or her tongue on the buccal aspect of the upper first molars
- he or she has a speech impediment which may be related to the fraenum
- the fraenum is causing trauma or is being traumatized.

Pressure from parents to intervene at an early age should be resisted since a number of prominent lingual fraena regress with age.

Pericision

Pericision is a technique used to reduce the amount of relapse following de-rotation of a single tooth. It is simply performed by using a number 15 blade to cut through the periodontal fibres attached to the coronal aspect of the root. The cut is made all the way round so that, in theory, the whole of the periodontal tissue can reattach itself in a better orientated position.

Pericision used to be extremely popular but many orthodontists now favour implementing longer-term retention, rather than intervening surgically with a technique which has not been fully proven.

Surgery for unerupted or misplaced canines

Impacted maxillary canines are amongst the most common of the eruption abnormalities, affecting some 3% of the population. Impaction may occur for a variety of reasons, including crowding, small lateral incisors, and the abnormal developmental position of the tooth germ (see Chapters 6 and 8). Maxillary canines particularly have a long path of eruption and during this process may be deflected. Palatal displacement is much more common than buccal displacement in the maxilla although the opposite is true in the mandible.

The failure to identify unerupted canines at an early age is one of the main problems with regard to their management. Their progress should be followed from about the age of 10 years and surgical intervention should be considered from 13–14 years of age. An attempt should always be made to localize the teeth clinically by palpation and radiographically (see Chapter 19) in order to assess any bucco-lingual displacement.

In addition, radiographs should be examined for:

- resorption of incisor roots (especially maxillary laterals)
- cystic change/enlargement of the follicle

- apical dilaceration
- displacement of related teeth.

Treatment planning must be based not only on a correct diagnosis but also on the wishes of the patient since orthodontic treatment options involving impacted canines may be long and demanding. In general terms, therefore, the options are:

- leave alone
- surgical exposure alone
- surgical exposure plus orthodontics
- extraction and discard the tooth (with or without replacement)
- surgically reposition
- auto-transplantation.

Non-intervention may be recommended in adults or older teenagers if the canine is asymptomatic, with no evidence or likelihood of any pathology (infection, cystic change or resorption) and no other orthodontics is required. If a decision is made to leave the tooth *in situ* it should be reviewed periodically to ensure that no pathology is developing.

Exposure of a tooth can be undertaken if:

- the canine is favourably positioned with its apex close to the correct position
- the potential path of eruption is not obstructed
- adequate space is available (or potentially available) to accommodate the canine.

Teeth that are situated buccally or in a mid-alveolar position, should be exposed by means of an apically repositioned flap (Figure 20.1). The surgical technique

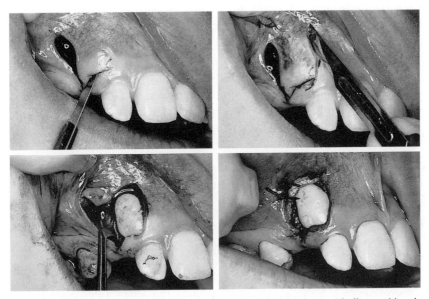

Figure 20.1 Surgical exposure of a labially located maxillary canine using an apically repositioned flap technique. Note how the attached keratinized mucosa has fitted around the neck of the tooth

of the apically repositioned flap generally results in a better appearance, providing a sound gingival margin with an attached, keratinized mucosa, which resists inflammation and maintains the depth of the labial sulcus. It also has other added advantages in that dressings are not needed and the dento-gingival attachment created helps to prevent marginal bone loss and gingival recession.

Palatally situated teeth should be exposed by removing a 'lid' of tissue over the crown of the tooth. Any bone covering the crown of the tooth should be carefully removed, taking particular care not to damage the crown of the tooth or the adjacent roots. Because of the phenomenal ability of the palatal mucosa to regrow, the exposure is usually kept open by stitching a pack into position – normally comprised of 1 cm ribbon gauze soaked in compound iodoform paint (Whitehead's varnish), as in Figure 20.2 or by use of an acrylic plate.

As long as the crown of the tooth is near the coronal third of the adjacent teeth, simple exposure is usually all that is required to encourage a tooth to erupt. However, for teeth which are more deeply placed, it may be advisable to attach a bracket onto the palatal aspect of the unerupted crown, a procedure which is often complicated by the presence of blood and saliva. Very deep canines should have a special bracket with a gold chain attached. In such cases a flap may be raised and replaced without removing much palatal tissue. Orthodontic, sub-mucosal traction can then be applied to bring the tooth into the mouth prior to further fixed appliance therapy. The techniques are usually successful but somewhat prolonged, 18–24 months being an average time to complete treatment. Frequently, compromises have to be made, however, and the retention of deciduous canines, space closure following extraction of the canine, and even implants should be considered (see below).

A decision to extract and discard a canine should never be undertaken lightly

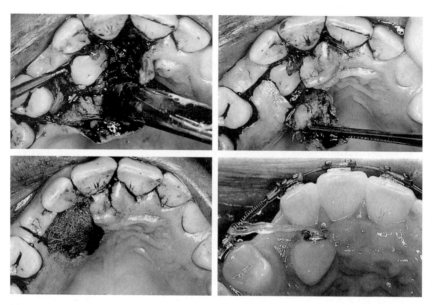

Figure 20.2 Surgical exposure of a palatally located maxillary canine (see text for explanation)

but there are some occasions when this is a preferred line of treatment. Such occasions would include:

- cases with totally excluded canines and a good lateral incisor-premolar contact
- cases where a canine is so far displaced that there is little other option
- cases in whom active resorption of adjacent roots can be demonstrated.

Even in cases of resorbing lateral incisors, however, there are times when it may be preferable to extract the incisor to allow eruption of the canine.

When a tooth has been extracted, there may be occasions when the space created has to be replaced by some means. Three alternatives are available:

- provision of a removable prosthesis (denture)
- provision of a fixed prosthesis (bridge)
- replacement by osseointegrated implant.

The use of implants has grown markedly during the last 20 years and shows no sign of abating. Ingenious uses of implants in relation to orthodontic treatment have also included the use of fixtures for providing anchorage in fixed appliance therapy. (The details of such treatment are outside the scope of this book but can be found in the relevant literature.)

In carefully selected cases, where there are no medical contraindications, it is possible to undertake surgical repositioning or reimplantation/transplantation of the canine, thereby avoiding the need for either future prosthetic replacement or possibly a prolonged course of orthodontic treatment. Despite their similar objectives, the two techniques are completely different.

Surgical repositioning is a one-stage technique of moving the tooth crown whilst maintaining the apical position in order to try to maintain pulp vitality (Figure 20.3). The crown can be moved in a fairly wide arc but providing the apical displacement is small, the blood supply should remain intact and thereby avoid pulp necrosis. Unlike transplantation the tooth is not removed from its socket. Success in surgical movement of teeth with incompletely formed roots is attributed to the rich vascularity of the apical region and the presence of undifferentiated mesenchymal tissue in the remnant of the dental papilla. This permits the vascular supply needed to repair severed or torn tissues. The technique is limited by the availability of space, the degree of root maturation (ideally half to two-thirds of root is formed) and the degree of tooth rotation about the apex that is required. Postoperatively the vitality of the tooth should be evaluated periodically.

Transplantation, however, is a technique whereby a tooth is reimplanted after removal into a modified or newly created socket (Figure 20.4). As in repositioning, sufficient space must be available (both mesiodistally and verti-cally). Various success rates have been quoted for transplantation but success is more likely when the root apex is wide open and the socket has been created with minimal trauma. Excessive instrumentation during elevation or damage to the tooth with a bur also increases the likelihood of failure. Generally, root canal therapy should not be attempted at the time of transplantation; instead, the need for this should be assessed after the tooth has been stabilized. It is the current view that transplanted teeth should be root filled after dressing with calcium hydroxide during the three months following surgery in order to minimize the tendency to root resorption. If this procedure is left until signs of resorption are

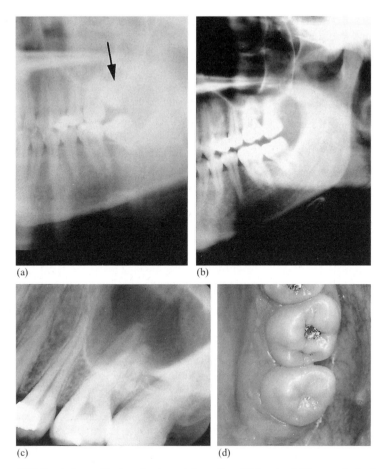

(a)   (b)

(c)   (d)

Figure 20.3 Surgical repositioning of an impacted maxillary third molar. (a) Preoperatively; (b, c) three years postoperatively; (d) clinical appearance with healthy gingivae

apparent on a radiograph, the long-term prognosis for the transplanted tooth is said to be much poorer (as so often, however, there are few well-controlled clinical trials to validate this).

In order to minimize the likelihood of ankylosis, at the time of operation the repositioned or transplanted tooth should not be rigidly splinted. Partial or total pulp obliteration may occur following either procedure, and root resorption is more common in transplanted teeth, invariably occurring at the cervical margin due to the gripping, with an instrument, of the tooth in this area. Continuing root development is an indication of revascularization and confirmation of a good prognosis. Nevertheless, it should again be emphasized that transplantation of teeth should only be carried out when orthodontic alignment is clearly contraindicated.

Surgery for other unerupted or misplaced teeth
Other impacted teeth are encountered from time to time. Upper incisors occasionally require surgical exposure to facilitate their eruption. The criteria

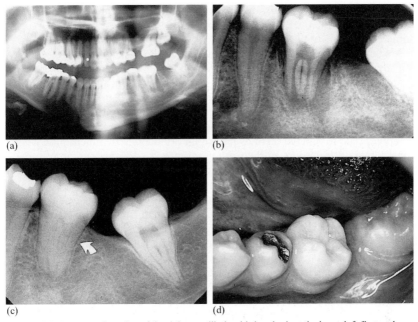

(a)   (b)

(c)   (d)

Figure 20.4 Autotransplantation of the right mandibular third molar into the lower left first molar socket. (a, b) Immediate postoperative stage; (c, d) two years postoperatively. Note the bone healing around the transplanted tooth with the formation of lamina dura (arrow). Also note the partial pulp obliteration

are similar to the surgical exposure of labially placed canines. The failure of eruption is often associated with the presence of a supernumerary tooth obstructing the path of eruption of the incisor. In such cases, provided that the timing is right, the space for eruption is adequate, and the position of the incisor is favourable, it will often erupt following removal of the supernumerary tooth. Provided that the incisor is not too high, an apically repositioned flap is appropriate. If, following exposure, the tooth still fails to erupt, then traction may be applied to bring the incisor down into the line of the arch. Where the incisor is more poorly positioned (as may be the case with a dilacerated incisor resulting from trauma to the deciduous incisors), it is usually very high and not palpable, a gold chain may be bonded in a similar fashion to that described for the maxillary canine. This facilitates submucosal traction to draw the tooth down until it is beneath the attached gingiva, at which time it will either break through on its own or will require a small exposure. Unerupted central incisors should not be exposed in the non-attached mucosa, since a very poor gingival contour will result and the long-term prognosis for the periodontium is poor.

When fully erupted and correctly positioned, the third molars may form an important part of a normally functioning occlusion. Third molars should be removed when there is a valid clinical indication. However, impaction of lower third molars is a common problem (see Chapter 9). There is no convincing evidence that impacted lower third molars cause lower incisor imbrication although some evidence exists that they may aggravate it. On occasion however, third molar removal may be justified as part of an active orthodontic treatment plan. Occasionally, a mildly mesio-angularly impacted third molar may be uprighted orthodontically or even surgically, usually as part of a simple adjunctive treatment plan.

Many of the orthodontic aspects associated with supernumerary teeth have already been discussed in Chapters 6 and 8. If a supernumerary tooth is symptomless and deeply buried, it is generally best to leave it *in situ* but to review its position from time to time. In other cases it is appropriate to arrange removal of a buried supernumerary tooth. This might be indicated if, for example, there are signs of any pathology such as cyst formation. It would also be appropriate to remove them as part of an orthodontic treatment plan when a supernumerary tooth was in the way of any proposed orthodontic tooth movement. If removal is planned, then accurate localization is absolutely essential prior to any surgical procedure although the vast majority of unerupted supernumeraries displace palatally. In addition, surgery should be delayed where possible until the root formation of the adjacent teeth is nearing completion (see Chapters 6 and 19).

In most cases, taking into account the age of the patient and the difficulty of access, these teeth are often best removed under general anaesthesia, usually on a day-case basis. The surgical approach depends upon their position and the same principles apply as with removal of unerupted canine teeth. It must be stressed that a minimum of bone should be removed to gain access to the supernumerary tooth and that great care should be taken not to damage the standing permanent teeth. Exposure of any unerupted normal incisors and interference with their follicles should generally be avoided since this may lead to the formation of scar tissue, which in itself can impede eruption and so necessitate a later procedure to uncover the incisor.

The impaction of other teeth is less common but not rare. It may affect lower canines and upper and lower premolars especially, and each case must be assessed individually. However, the principles for management are largely the same as those of the impacted maxillary canine (see above) although, since they are commonly displaced due to a lack of space, extraction of such teeth is more common than with maxillary canines.

Retained roots may also interfere with orthodontic tooth movement and it is important that 'routine' extractions are carried out carefully, the roots of the delivered tooth being inspected closely for signs of fracture. Should a fractured root be discovered it is important to extract it with minimal bone removal, preferably by opening a window in the buccal plate (being careful to avoid damage to the roots of adjacent teeth), thereby preserving the height of the alveolus.

Surgery on hard tissues

Surgical procedures are occasionally undertaken on the bony tissues as an adjunct to orthodontic treatment. Minor procedures are relatively uncommon although occasionally a pathological process, such as fibrous dysplasia, requires the removal of hard tissues. In addition the formation of odontomes, the development of submerged teeth or areas of sclerotic bone may require minor oral surgery.

Finally mention should also be made of the surgical procedures which are carried out in relation to orthognathic and cleft surgery. This may include bone grafting, sectioning of the palate to aid maxillary expansion, and other dento-alveolar procedures which are discussed later in this text. In all cases the purpose of treatment should be to facilitate the end result – one of a contented patient who is pleased with a good aesthetic and functional result.

Further reading

Sailer, H.F. and Pajarola, G.F. (1999). *Oral Surgery for the General Dentist*. New York: Thieme.

Chapter 21

Orthodontic treatment in the adult

The adult patient in comparison to the child

Before discussing the orthodontic options available to adult patients it would seem worthwhile to define exactly what we mean by an '*adult*' in the orthodontic context. An adult patient is one in whom growth has ceased to be of relevance in the treatment planning for the correction of a malocclusion. For the purposes of the current discussion this would usually mean a patient older than 16 years. This does not mean that there is no growth after this age. Indeed, recent evidence would suggest small, but significant, increments of growth affecting the facial form occur into the thirties or perhaps even later. However, such growth is unlikely to cause any significant change in the skeletal pattern or soft tissue profile of the face over the relative short term of an active treatment. It is also unlikely that such small increments of growth occurring over a long period of time would be of any assistance in the correction of the malocclusion. For example, both extra-oral traction (headgear) and functional appliances would be of limited use in any adult treatment.

Treatment planning

There is a traditional belief amongst many clinicians that orthodontic manage-ment of the adult is more difficult than that of the child. This is not necessarily true. The treatment need not be any more difficult provided it is recognized that the treatment planning of these cases needs careful attention, and that several additional factors need consideration at the outset.

Past examination of UK national statistics (Dental Practice Board) would suggest that adult treatments, in general, fail more frequently than those for children, thus reinforcing the belief that orthodontic treatment in this group is more complex. However, such statistics probably reflect more the inappropriate use of simple removable appliances, since in most adult treatments a fixed appliance should constitute the 'standard' contemporary approach.

In fact there are certain advantages in treating this group of patients, the principal one being the ability of the adult to clearly identify the aesthetic or even the functional problem; these patients usually have a far better perception of their malocclusion than does the child (see McKiernan *et al.*, 1992). However, although this type of patient may play a role in deciding treatment goals, it is equally important that their contribution be restricted when it comes to selection of the appliance system. Frequently, it is patient pressure that has led to inappropriate selection of a removable appliance in the past.

Some of the main advantages and disadvantages of treating the adult as opposed to the child patient are listed below.

Advantages
1. The facial form and skeletal pattern is largely established. Unfavourable growth during treatment is not a factor.
2. The patient is usually able to identify clearly the aesthetic problem.
3. This type of patient usually has excellent compliance. There is often an element of self-referral and the patient is strongly internally motivated.
4. Since growth is largely complete, orthognathic surgery may be included in any immediate treatment plan where the skeletal or profile discrepancy is to be corrected.

Disadvantages
1. Treatment cannot depend on the assistance of favourable growth. Appliances that depend on such growth for the majority of the correction have only limited use (e.g. headgear or functionals).
2. The adult patient is likely to be more demanding when it comes to assessing the final result.
3. There can be a problem with social acceptability of fixed appliances for adults in some environments. The improved appearance of the new generation of aesthetic tooth-coloured (or clear) brackets helps to solve this problem. In selected cases lingually bonded, fixed appliances may also improve the aesthetics.
4. Dento-alveolar camouflage of underlying skeletal problems is only usually appropriate in the milder discrepancies. In the adult patient, greater consideration needs to be given to the effects on the profile of the soft tissues following tooth movement. This is especially true where overjet reduction is being planned.
5. There are often also greater repercussions on the surrounding tissues; for example, ulceration may be a short-term result of fixed appliances whilst root resorption might be a longer-term consequence.
6. There is often slower initial movement of the teeth in the adult. Once the turnover of the cells in the periodontal ligament has increased, tooth movement speeds up.
7. There is usually more initial pain following an appliance adjustment in the adult. Such discomfort normally recedes after 3–4 days.

There are additional considerations involved in the process of treatment planning in the adult:

- having been 'around longer' the adult is more likely to present with retained roots, impactions, apical cysts and other local pathologies
- previous loss of permanent teeth, due to caries for instance, may leave spacing in the dental arch which is poorly placed to assist in the occlusal correction
- there may be areas of significant apical root resorption which could prejudice planned tooth movement

- existing or previous periodontal disease may limit the amount and duration of possible tooth movement
- there may be a history of temporomandibular joint pain which orthodontics could worsen, at least in the short term
- there may be systemic disease present which might affect the treatment approach.

These points, along with others, would need to be addressed prior to commencing any treatment. Any active periodontal disease should be treated and stabilized, whilst restorations in the teeth should be made sound at the same time that active caries is treated.

In the situation where significant and inappropriate spacing in the dental arches is present, bridgework and/or dental implants may often be a valuable addition to any plan. Conversely, pre-existing bridgework or crowns/veneers may need to be removed to allow orthodontic correction.

In addition to these general points, careful thought also needs to be given to the likely active treatment span: over-ambitious tooth movements should either be restricted or avoided altogether. Decisions on extractions may be dictated by the prognosis of the standing teeth; nonetheless some consideration should also be given to the difficulty that can arise in adults when attempting to close excessive extraction space.

In the adult a perfect occlusal result is not always possible, the treatment goal being determined by a process similar to Figure 21.1.

In developing such a treatment goal, the aesthetic correction requested by the patient is an important consideration. The patient would also expect this goal to be achieved within a reasonable time scale. As an example, our patients are usually told to expect 20–24 months of active appliance therapy.

The result will also be determined by the presenting pathology (missing teeth, loss of alveolar bone, etc.), but the eventual goal should also be a functioning occlusion – an important factor in the stability of the final result.

In the achievement of a good static and functioning post-treatment occlusion it must be remembered that post-treatment 'settling in' cannot be depended upon in the adult as it might be in the child. Therefore the occlusion must be precisely detailed to a conclusion, another good reason for using a fixed appliance.

A 'set-up' as shown in Figure 21.2 is often helpful in deciding the eventual occlusal goal; the various options for tooth movement being rehearsed on the study casts.

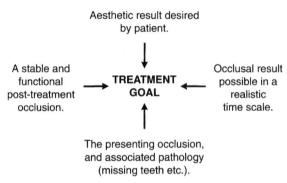

Figure 21.1 Establishing the treatment goal

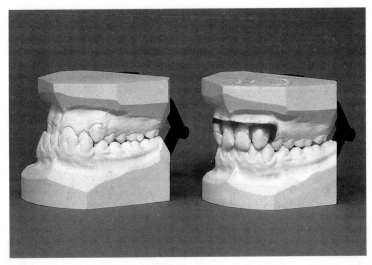

Figure 21.2 A 'set-up' of planned tooth and jaw movements. This is achieved by sectioning then repositioning the study casts

Treatment

The treatment of adult malocclusion falls into two main categories (Proffit, 2000):

1. Comprehensive treatment – achieving the best functional and aesthetic occlusion possible:

   (a) by dental alveolar movements with an orthodontic appliance
   (b) by orthognathic surgery in combination with orthodontic movements.

2. Adjunctive treatment – accepting the overall arrangement of the teeth but making local tooth movements to improve the occlusion whilst making it both more functional and more physiological. This could involve inter-speciality treatment, for example bridgework.

Comprehensive treatment

This involves full correction of the malocclusion to the best possible aesthetic and functional occlusion. In mild to moderate malocclusions with only a limited skeletal discrepancy this can be best achieved by applying a fully fixed preadjusted appliance (see Chapter 17) from second molar to second molar to achieve a good dento-alveolar correction (Figure 21.3). However, since appliances which rely on growth modification (see Chapter 18) are inappropriate in the adult, greater care should be paid to the facial profile, and a combination of orthodontics and surgery will need to be considered in patients with any significant degree of presenting skeletal discrepancy (see Chapter 22).

The treatment time for both dento-alveolar and orthognathic approaches will be similar as will the appliance used. This will usually be fixed, with the

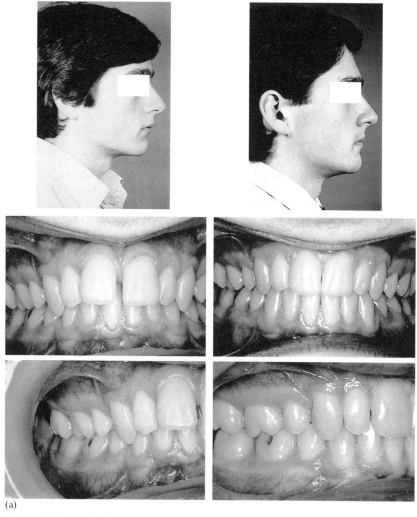

(a)

Figure 21.3 Comprehensive treatment of a malocclusion in the adult patient using a preadjusted fixed appliance. (a) Start and finish; (b) mechanics employed

occasional assistance of an upper removable to allow clearance of occlusal interferences during the early stages of treatment.

Removable appliances as the sole system for comprehensive correction of malocclusion are usually inappropriate in the adult for a number of reasons:

1. They are poorly worn due to slow adjustment to the immediate effects on speech and eating.
2. They do not move teeth with sufficient precision to achieve regularly the desired standard of occlusal finish.
3. They are not, consistently, clinically effective in adults.
4. There is only limited post-treatment settling in such patients.
5. They reduce overbite by relative intrusion from an anterior bite plane (see

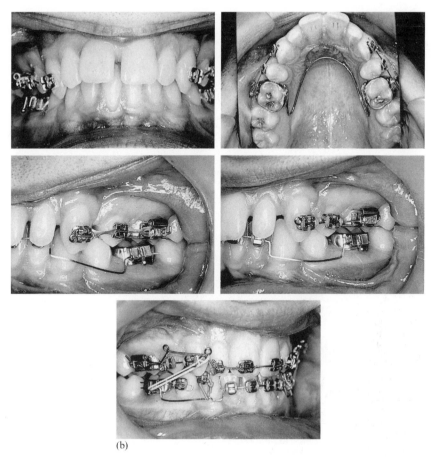

(b)

Figure 21.3 (*continued*)

Chapter 16). This is an inappropriate approach in the adult where true intrusion of lower incisors is usually preferred. In any event, bite planes are a much less effective approach in the non-growing adult.

6. They are biomechanically less efficient since ageing changes to the alveolar bone and periodontium will increase the tendency of teeth to tip.

Adjunctive treatment

Where removable appliances may have more of a role is in adjunctive treatments in which limited, usually localized, tooth movements are undertaken to achieve a more physiological and functional occlusion. Such treatments are often associated with other dental procedures, for example advanced restorative or periodontal treatments, the aim being to improve the dental health or function without necessarily achieving an ideal, or indeed Class I, occlusal result, which would require the comprehensive approach, previously described (see Figures 21.5 and 21.6).

Figure 17.8 demonstrates a typical adjunctive treatment where a removable

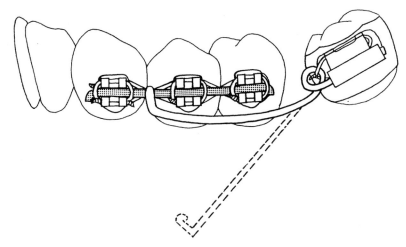

Figure 21.4 Example of an adjunctive type of treatment where a molar is to be uprighted prior to bridgework being placed mesial to it

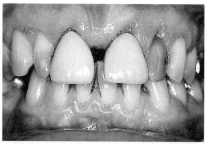

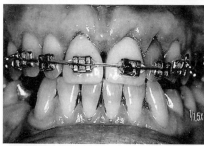

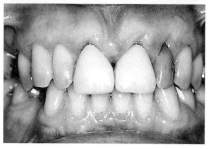

Figure 21.5 Example of an adjunctive treatment where previously periodontally involved and splayed incisors are being brought together, by means of a simple fixed appliance, prior to placement of a splint retainer. (Note the enlarged porcelain crowns on the central incisors – this was a previous, purely restorative solution reducing the diastema)

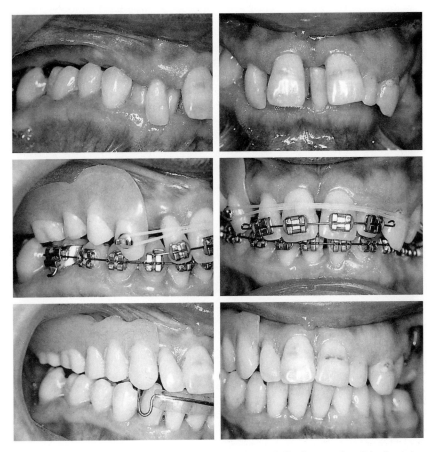

Figure 21.6 Example of an adult treatment which is on the borderline between the adjunctive and comprehensive type. The patient's initial presentation is shown at the top. Numerous teeth are missing, there is a large displacement on closure with a traumatic bite such that a denture cannot be comfortably worn. In addition the patient is experiencing temporomandibular joint symptoms. In the treatment views note the upper partial denture being used as an anchor whilst the overjet is being reduced. As a consequence, the incisor spacing (due originally to loss of periodontal support through disease) has been closed. The bottom views show the finished occlusion in retainers prior to the definitive restorative work being commenced

appliance has been used to bring a canine crown from its palatal position, eliminating a displacement on closure. Figure 21.4 shows a more conventional treatment where a molar has been uprighted and a plunger cusp mechanism eliminated prior to placement of a crown.

Finally, Figure 21.5 shows a patient in whom splayed incisors have been collected together following the stabilization of the causative factor (chronic periodontal disease), the management of a similar, although more complex problem is shown in Figure 21.6.

Conclusion

Adult orthodontics is a fast growing area of the speciality. In the USA prior to 1970 this group represented 5% of all orthodontic patients. In the 1980s this was estimated to have risen to 20–25% of treatments. One may speculate that during 2000–2010 it is likely in the Western world that approximately 40% of orthodontic patients presenting for treatment will be over 16 years of age. Many of the treatments will be of an interspeciality nature.

When adults are treated, initial tooth movement may be slower and more painful than in the child or adolescent. However, adult patients are generally highly motivated and, if planned with expertise, may be treated to a finished result of a consistently high standard.

Further reading

Kiyak, H.A. and Bell, R. (1991). Psychological considerations in surgery and orthodontics. In *Surgical Orthodontic Treatment* (W.R. Proffit and R.P. White, eds). St Louis: Mosby Yearbook.

McKiernan, E.X.F., Jones, M.L. and McKiernan, F. (1992). Psychological profiles and motives of adult patients seeking orthodontic treatment. *International Journal of Adult Orthodontics and Orthognathic Surgery*, **3**, 187–98.

Proffit, W.R. (2000). Adjunctive treatment for adults (Chapter 20, pp. 616–43); Special considerations in comprehensive treatment of adults (Chapter 21, pp. 644–73). In *Contemporary Orthodontics*. St Louis: Mosby Yearbook.

Proffit, W.R., Phillips, C. and Dann, C. (1994). Who seeks surgicial-orthodontic treatment? *International Journal of Adult Orthodontics and Orthognathic Surgery*, **5**, 153–60.

Vanarsdall, R.L. and Musich, D.R. (1985). Adult orthodontics: diagnosis and treatment. In *Orthodontics, Current Principles and Techniques*. (T.M. Graber and B.F. Swain, eds). St Louis: Mosby Yearbook.

Chapter 22

The role of orthognathic surgery: planning and treatment

Planning and treatment

The surgical correction of jaw deformity aims to create 'straight jaws', a literal definition of the word 'orthognathic'. Such corrections are largely achieved by osteotomies, a surgical technique by which parts of the jaw are sectioned and then moved into new positions whilst preserving their blood supply.

Although commonly indicated for moderate to severe skeletal discrepancies of the Class II or Class III type, these procedures also allow the correction of vertical discrepancies (long or short faces), open bite deformities, transverse discrepancies (asymmetries) and congenital craniofacial syndromes (e.g. cleft lip and palate, first arch deformities or the craniosynostoses). Except in severe syndromal cases, definitive surgery is usually delayed until around the age of 16 years, when most maxillary and mandibular growth of any significance has occurred (see Chapter 3).

Patient complaints

Patients often present to orthodontists and dental surgeons complaining of the appearance of their teeth. Concerns about their facial appearance and speech are volunteered less frequently but are often present and may provide a further underlying cause for concern to the patient. Therefore, a careful history is important in such cases. It is always important to explore the patient's motivation for seeking treatment and to emphasize that orthognathic surgery is an elective procedure. The clinician should never try to persuade the patient to undergo treatment but rather should respond to their concerns. A careful explanation of what can be done should be given and it is an advantage if written and/or visual material, weighing potential advantages and disadvantages, can be given to the patient so that a carefully considered, informed decision may be made.

Documentation

Standard records should include:

- a detailed description of the patients' concerns
- facial and dental photographs
- dental study casts usually based in centric occlusion

- an orthopantomogram (OPT) and lateral cephalogram, with a postero-anterior (PA) cephalogram for those patients presenting with an asymmetry
- a detailed dental history and examination
- a detailed medical history and examination.

Occasionally, a speech assessment will be required and, in complex syndromes, three-dimensional radiographic techniques (e.g. 3D computerized tomography reformats – see Chapter 19) can be valuable.

Analysis

This needs to be based on:

1. A detailed clinical assessment of dento-facial form, dimensions and relation-ships (Figure 22.1a).
2. A lateral cephalometric analysis for all antero-posterior and vertical discre-pancies (Figure 22.1b).

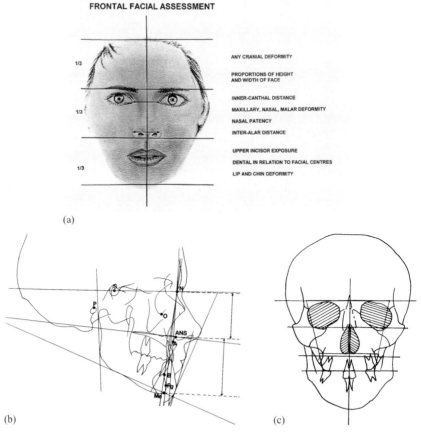

Figure 22.1 (a) The frontal clinical assessment. (b) The lateral cephalometric assessment. (c) The postero-anterior (PA) cephalometric assessment

3. PA cephalometric analysis for asymmetries (Figure 22.1c).
4. A comparison of traced lateral cephalogram films with standard skull templates of the appropriate age and racial group (e.g. Bolton standards).

By following such a regime, usually a clear diagnosis can be made. For example, in Figure 22.2 the patient shown has vertical excess and an antero-posterior deficiency of the maxilla, with an antero-posterior excess of the mandible and vertical excess of the chin. In addition, there is significant natural dento-alveolar compensation for the underlying skeletal discrepancy with, in particular, retroclination of lower incisors acting to disguise the underlying mandibular excess (Figure 22.3a).

The presence of any medical conditions or dental problems which may interfere with surgery or orthodontics should be considered at an early stage in the planning.

Presurgical orthodontics

The usual aims of orthodontic treatment prior to surgery are to eliminate any dento-alveolar compensation (and thus reveal the true jaw discrepancy) and create coordinated, well-aligned dental arches, which will be compatible with each other after surgery. This presurgical orthodontic phase facilitates the planned skeletal and facial correction.

In patients presenting with a severe Class III problem the lower incisors are commonly retroclined (Figure 22.4). These pretreatment tooth positions naturally act to 'compensate' and 'camouflage' the original deformity. Presurgical orthodontic correction (see shaded teeth in Figure 22.4) serves to reveal the 'true' jaw discrepancy and thus permits full correction of the facial skeleton by means of the subsequent surgery.

In Class II cases, the dento-alveolar compensation presents typically as shown in Figure 22.4 (Division 1 and Division 2 cases) but often these different presentations of Class II require similar surgical corrections. In all cases, a decision needs to be made on whether the planned orthodontic treatment requires tooth extraction within the dental arch to facilitate the necessary tooth movement. Such a decision will depend on the need for space and will also be related to the extent of the crowding present. In general, poorly positioned ectopic teeth should be removed.

Once the orthodontic treatment aims have been achieved, large-sized rectangular archwires (usually a minimum of 0.19×0.25 in) will need to be placed. At least six weeks should be allowed for these wires to become passive retainers of the tooth positions. Immediately prior to surgery, 'surgical hooks' should be attached to the archwire (or the brackets) to aid surgical intermaxillary fixation and/or postsurgical elastic traction.

Planning

Due to the many changes, including those related to growth, that occur during orthodontic preparation, detailed surgical planning will usually be delayed until the last few weeks prior to surgery. It should be based primarily on a sound clinical analysis.

Some form of detailed planning, based principally on lateral cephalometric

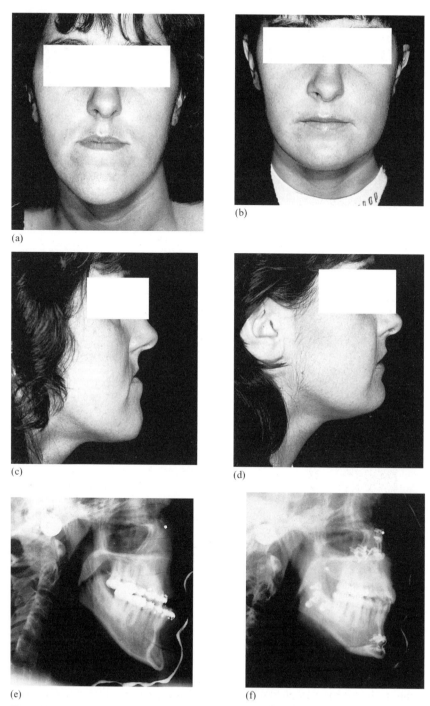

Figure 22.2 (a, c) A patient with a Class III (horizontal and vertical) orthognathic problem at presentation. (b, d) The appearance of the face after orthodontic and surgical correction. (c, f) The surgical change achieved shown by pre- and postsurgical cephalograms

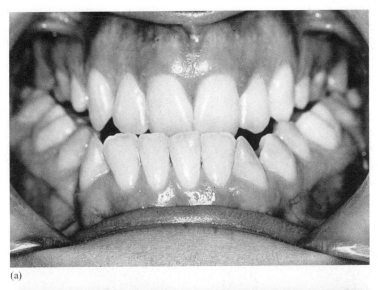

(a)

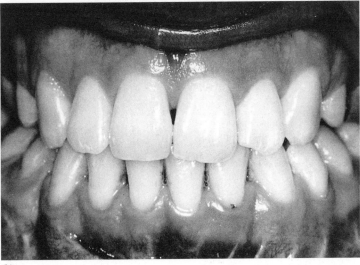

(b)

Figure 22.3 (a, b) Pretreatment occlusion and the occlusal correction achieved after orthodontics and surgery (same patient as Figure 22.2). (Orthodontic treatment performed by Mr R. Samuels).

tracing, is usually appropriate in the attempt to quantify the intended movements of the bones. Such a process may be performed manually by cutting and adjusting multiple tracings. However, this is a tedious process and simple inexpensive computer programs are now available which allow different movements to be rehearsed quickly on-screen. Figure 22.5 shows such an analysis performed for the patient in Figure 22.2. In the average case such systems can be surprisingly accurate (see Eales *et al.*, 1994). The result of the planned facial profile change can also be clearly shown to the patient through the adjustment

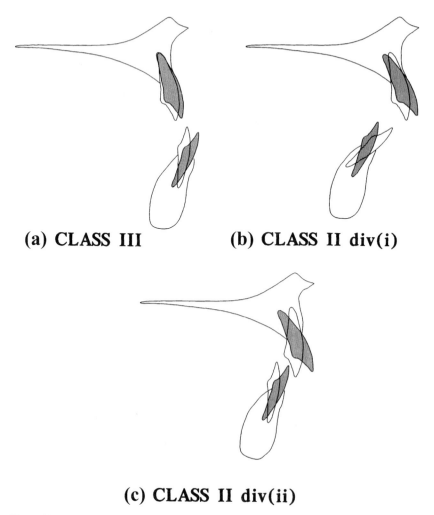

(a) CLASS III   **(b) CLASS II div(i)**

(c) CLASS II div(ii)

Figure 22.4 (a–c) The most commonly presenting incisor position, which naturally serves to camouflage the underlying skeletal discrepancy. This is shown for three presenting malocclusions. The shaded teeth show the tooth movements (orthodontic decompensation) achieved prior to surgery

of digitized presurgical photographs of the patient. This technique is termed 'video planning' and again provides a surprisingly accurate prediction of the results of both tooth and jaw movements.

These planned movements are then translated to articulated dental study casts in the laboratory using reference lines to measure distances. When a maxillary procedure is planned, the models are usually placed on an anatomical semi-adjustable articulator. Occlusal wafers/splints are constructed (in acrylic) in the final and (in two-jaw bimaxillary surgery cases) intermediate surgical positions to facilitate accurate location of the jaws at the time of operation.

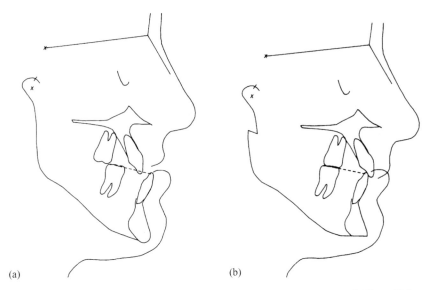

(a)   (b)

Figure 22.5 (a) A computer-generated lateral cephalometric analysis of the patient in Figure 22.2. (b) Using the same software (in this instance COG 3.1), a profile prediction tracing, taking into account orthodontic and surgical effects, is generated

Mid-face surgery

Le Fort 1 osteotomy

Le Fort 1 Osteotomy (Figure 22.6a) is the most versatile, stable and commonly used of all orthognathic procedures. It permits the repositioning of the upper jaw in all dimensions and, if necessary, the maxilla can be divided into multiple segments. The key to success is to create an ideal position of the upper incisor teeth in relation to the upper lip with their centre line on the facial centre. The antero-posterior discrepancy of the jaws is fully corrected. This will produce an ideal naso-labial angle and a good lip profile. The desired occlusal plane is created by vertical posterior movements and, in anterior open bite cases, posterior intrusion (maxillary rotation) permits full correction.

A sulcus incision from first molar to first molar allows exposure of the entire anterior maxilla, which is sectioned with surgical saws and osteotomes along the anterior wall, tuberosity, lateral nasal wall and septum. It is then digitally 'down-fractured' and mobilized with forceps. The bone is pedicled on the soft tissues laterally and palatally. Bony interferences can then be removed, intermaxillary fixation applied across the planned occlusal splint (acrylic wafer), and bone fixation with wires or (more commonly) plates and screws inserted. The post-operative use of intermaxillary fixation depends on the rigidity of the fixation and personal preference of the surgeon. In the author's experience, it can be avoided in 95% of cases.

Le Fort 2 osteotomy

Le Fort 2 osteotomies (Figure 22.6b) are valuable especially when there is a genuine antero-posterior (and sometimes vertical) deficiency of the nose and

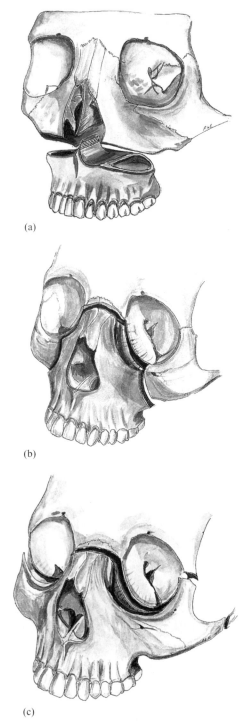

(a)

(b)

(c)

Figure 22.6 The most commonly employed maxillary osteotomies: (a) Le Fort 1 osteotomy; (b) Le Fort 2 osteotomy; (c) Le Fort 3 osteotomy

maxilla. When the whole mid-face is involved, including both cheekbones, a Le Fort 3 osteotomy (Figure 22.6c) is required. These procedures can sometimes be combined with Le Fort 1 osteotomies in more complex cases.

Premaxillary osteotomy

Premaxillary osteotomies (Wassmund, Wunderer or down-fracture techniques) are segmental procedures which used to be very popular. Modern fixed band orthodontic treatment ensures that they are now rarely indicated.

Mandibular surgery

Sagittal split osteotomy

This is the mandibular equivalent of the Le Fort 1. Although first described by Trauner and Obwegeser in 1957, the modification of Dal Pont (1961) is the procedure most commonly carried out (Figure 22.7a). By splitting the outer part of the ramus from the inner, it permits the entire tooth-bearing part of the

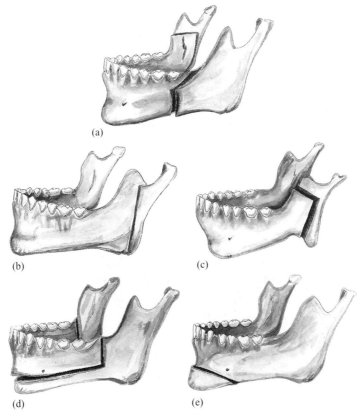

(a)

(b)   (c)

(d)   (e)

Figure 22.7 The most commonly employed mandibular osteotomies. (a) Sagittal split osteotomy of mandible. (b) Sub-sigmoid osteotomy of mandibular ramus. (c) Inverted L osteotomy of mandibular ramus. (d) Total sub-apical osteotomy of mandible. (e) Genioplasty

mandible to be repositioned anteriorly or posteriorly. It is carried out through an oral approach and can be fixed with screws (often inserted through a small transbuccal skin incision), plates and screws, or wire.

Its versatility is slightly restricted by the need to avoid lengthening the ramus against masticatory and supra-hyoid muscle pull since this may prove unstable. Advancements tend to be less stable than posterior movements but there is some evidence that screw fixation and supra-hyoid myotomy improve stability in such cases.

Sub-sigmoid osteotomy

Sub-sigmoid osteotomy (Figure 22.7b) of the mandibular ramus was once the most popular technique to correct prognathism and used to be carried out by an extra-oral approach. The procedure can now be performed intra-orally but it tends to be technically difficult to fix the bones by such a process and may prove less stable than the equivalent sagittal split osteotomy. A further disadvantage is that intermaxillary fixation is usually required.

Inverted L osteotomy

Inverted L osteotomies (Figure 22.7c) are indicated when the ramus must be lengthened and advanced (e.g. first arch deformity, condylar hypoplasia). They are usually carried out from an external approach with bone grafts inserted into the spaces created.

Sub-apical osteotomy

Sub-apical osteotomies are indicated when only the tooth-bearing part of the mandible needs to be moved. Although usually anterior segments are set up or down, the entire dental arch can be repositioned if desired (total sub-apical osteotomy, Figure 22.7d).

Body osteotomy

Body osteotomies may be valuable in severe prognathism and asymmetry, the cuts usually being made ideally in an edentulous area, interdentally or after extraction of teeth. The inferior dental nerve is protected.

Genioplasty

Genioplasty (Figure 22.7e) is probably the most valuable mandibular procedure of all, and is normally carried out by means of a horizontal sliding osteotomy. The chin can be advanced in one or two slices, with or without the addition of a bone graft. With appropriate bone removal or grafting the chin can be repositioned in any dimension. Widening and narrowing may also be performed. This simple operation often produces the most dramatic changes to the profile and overall appearance of the face.

Results and stability

Figures 22.2 and 22.3 show the changes achieved in the Class III case described earlier. Initial orthodontic decompensation has been performed by means of a fixed appliance (there is rarely a place for other than an Edgewise derived fixed appliance in such treatment). Surgical correction has been achieved by means of a maxillary advancement and intrusion at the Le Fort 1 level, a mandibular pushback by bilateral sagittal splits, and a vertical chin reduction genioplasty.

Figure 22.8 shows a Class II case where a significant profile improvement has

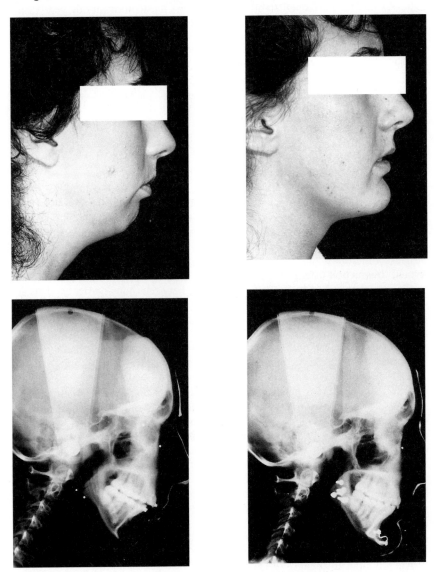

Figure 22.8 A patient presenting with a Class II Division 1 skeletal discrepancy where most of the profile improvement has been achieved by means of an advancement genioplasty

been achieved by means of a relatively small mandibular sagittal split advancement and a large genioplasty advancement. This demonstrates the value of the latter procedure, with a considerable change being obtained in the appearance of the face from this relatively minor procedure.

In almost every case, surgery is followed by a period of orthodontics (usually 3–6 months) to finalize tooth position and occlusion. Following the removal of the fixed appliance (debonding), conventional orthodontic retention is necessary (see Chapter 25). Patients undergoing orthognathic surgery are generally reviewed for a minimum of two years after surgery. Such audit of results indicates that the horizontal stability of a Le Fort 1 osteotomy at one year varies between 6 and 25% (depending on the study), with the vertical change more liable to relapse (16–45%). For sagittal split mandibular advancements, reported relapse at one year varies between 15 and 30%. The significance of reporting data at one year is that nearly all of the postsurgical skeletal relapse that is going to occur should have happened by that time. Not surprisingly, the long-term success of orthognathic treatment is very technique- and surgeon-sensitive.

Distraction osteogenesis

Osteotomies to reposition the jaws as described above have revolutionized the correction of dento-facial deformities. They are limited to some extent by the need to place the bones in a precise position at surgery, by the limitations on movements that this imposes, and by the enveloping soft tissues, which may be deficient. In addition, interventions during growth are usually avoided and bone grafts are sometimes required.

These limitations may be overcome, to some extent, by another technique, termed 'distraction osteogenesis' (DO), also known as 'callus distraction'. This is the 'mechanical induction of new bone between bony surfaces that are *gradually* pulled apart'. Although first described in long bones in 1905, the real pioneer in this field in orthopaedic surgery was Ilizarov working in Siberia (then in the USSR) from 1950 to 1990 and best known for leg lengthening. The method was not reported as applied to the mandible until published by McCarthy in 1992. Since then, devices which can move bone in one, two and several directions simultaneously have been described, some of which are external, some internal and yet others which are a combination of both. The method has also been applied to the mid-face and cranium and especially to congenital deformity.

The technique consists of making an osteotomy cut in the bone and attaching (by pins or screws in the bone, or fixation to teeth) a device which permits lengthening of the bone. After a latency period of a few days, this device or distracter is usually activated by turning a screw to produce small movements of lengthening of the bone (usually around one millimetre each day), and thus a gap in the bone forms. When the desired length has been achieved, the device is kept *in situ* for several weeks until bone has filled the gap. The device is then removed. At that stage, orthodontic support with a modified (prescription) functional appliance is often valuable.

The principal advantages of DO are:

1. The potential for interventions during growth.

2. The avoidance of the need for bone grafting in most cases.
3. The ability to lengthen the bone until the desired changes have been produced, limited to some extent by the device used and by biology.
4. The ability to lengthen previously grafted bone.
5. The ability to repeat DO if necessary at a later date.
6. The more minor surgery involved compared with conventional orthognathic surgery.
7. Simultaneous lengthening achieved of the soft-tissue matrix.

The principal disadvantages (at this time) are:

1. Scarring with external devices.
2. Length of distraction limitation with purely internal devices.
3. Difficulty in controlling direction.
4. The limitations of existing devices (although the number and variety of devices available are increasing rapidly).
5. Significant cooperation is required from both the patient and their family in most cases.

Without doubt, distraction osteogenesis is now revolutionizing the correction of skeletal facial deformity, especially in the management of severe congenital deformity in children.

Conclusion

Orthognathic surgery is very worthwhile in suitable cases. Although most surgery is by no means minor, three decades of surgical refinement of large numbers of cases have enabled it to become, in experienced hands, safe and effective. Both the orthodontics and surgery require careful planning. In addition, the overall treatment can take as long as 24 months. Therefore the patient needs to be highly motivated and their motivation for seeking treatment should be exhaustively explored by the clinicians concerned. Care should be taken to explain the planned changes in facial appearance to the patient. To assist in this process, systems which video capture images of the face have become available. Such images may then be adjusted by suitable software to rehearse the surgery and demonstrate the result to the patient. In more complex cases, three-dimensional plastic models (using data from 3D CT scans) can be constructed and the various surgical options rehearsed on the models in advance of operation.

Further reading

Eales, E.A., Newton, C., Jones, M.L. and Sugar, A. (1994). The accuracy of computerised prediction of the soft tissue profile. *International Journal of Adult Orthodontics and Orthognathic Surgery*, **9**, 141–52.

Grayson, B.H. and Santiago, P.E. (1999). Distraction osteogenesis. In *Seminars in Orthodontics*, Vol. 5 (P.L. Sadowsky, ed.), Part 1, pp. 1–58. Philadelphia: Saunders.

McCarthy, J.G., Schreiber, J., Karp, N. *et al.* (1992). Lengthening the human mandible by gradual distraction. *Journal of Plastic and Reconstructive Surgery*, **89**, 1–8.

Proffit, W.R. (2000). Combined surgical and orthodontic treatment. (Chapter 22, 674–709). In *Contemporary Orthodontics*. St Louis: Mosby Yearbook.

Sarver, D.M. (1996). Video cephalometric diagnosis: A new concept in treatment planning? *American Journal of Orthodontics and Dentofacial Orthopedics*, **109**, 128–36.

Sarver, D.M., Johnston, M.W. and Matukas, V.J. (1988). Video imaging for planning and counselling in orthognathic surgery. *Journal of Oral and Maxillofacial Surgery*, **46**, 939–45.

Sinclair, P.M. (1992). The long-term stability of orthognathic surgery. In *Stability and Relapse in Orthodontics*. (C. Burstone, ed.). Connecticut: Farmington.

Chapter 23

Orthodontic management of cleft lip and palate

Cleft lip with or without cleft palate is a highly visible congenital deformity of the mouth and face, and is a relatively common condition, occurring in approximately 1:700 live births in the Western world. There is some variation in incidence between racial groups. With modern ultrasonic scanning equipment it is usually possible to diagnose facial clefting from about the third month of pregnancy.

Aetiology

The cleft may be part of a syndrome or may occur in isolation. For some there is a clear familial history of facial clefting, implying a genetic disorder, but for the majority of cases the occurrence is sporadic, suggesting that as yet unidentified factors have an important role in the aetiology of the condition. However, this is an area of rapid development and the errors in the genetic messages that lead to the development of a cleft are only now beginning to be properly understood. Embryologically the nose, lip and primary palate are formed by the fusion of the medial nasal, lateral nasal and maxillary processes in about the 8th week of intrauterine life. Clefting may arise due to failure of fusion, or fusion followed by partial or total breakdown between the facial processes with continued facial growth. The secondary palate and soft palate fuse in the midline (with each other and with the nasal septum) during the 9th and 10th week and failure of fusion results in a cleft of the hard and/or soft palate (see Chapter 3).

Pierre Robin syndrome, in which there is a U-shaped cleft of the secondary palate, a retrusive mandible, and a risk of airway obstruction by the retro-positioned tongue in severe cases, is thought to arise due to the inability of the tongue to drop down from between the palatal shelves during palatogenesis.

Classification

There is no entirely satisfactory system of classification and this reflects the wide variety of presentation. For the individual patient it is probably most convenient just to describe the defect. However, for purposes of classification it is useful to divide clefts in three groups:

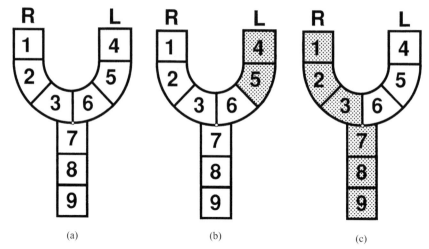

Figure 23.1 (a) A simple numerical classification system for clefts – the 'striped Y'. The lip is represented by 1 and 4; the alveolus by 2 and 5; the primary palate by 3 and 6; the hard palate by 7 and 8; and the soft palate by 9. (b) Left-sided cleft lip and alveolus only. (c) Right-sided complete cleft of lip and palate

1. Clefts of the primary palate – may involve only the lip, or the lip and alveolar process as far back as the incisive foramen.
2. Clefts of the secondary palate – may involve the soft palate only or the soft palate and hard palate as far forwards as the incisive foramen.
3. Clefts involving both the primary and secondary palate.

Clefts of the lip and primary palate may be unilateral (most commonly on the left side) or bilateral. In addition Kernahan (1971) has produced a symbolic method – the 'striped Y' to describe clefts (Figure 23.1). The small circle at the junction of the Y signifies the incisive foramen. This describes the extent of the cleft by cross-hatching the appropriate squares, and has the added advantage of lending itself to computerized records. In the UK all clefts are registered on a national database called CARE (Craniofacial Anomalies REgister). Other countries have similar central registration systems, which are essential to run a proper nationally coordinated system of care.

Effects of cleft lip and palate

Dental effects

Number of teeth. There may be missing teeth, extra teeth or the correct number of teeth. The area of the cleft is most frequently affected, but evidence is growing that there is a higher incidence of absent teeth elsewhere in the mouth, most especially in the second premolar regions of both dental arches.

Morphology of teeth. The lateral incisor on the cleft side may be diminutive and/or peg shaped.

Structure of teeth. There may be enamel hypoplasia and/or hypomineralization of teeth, especially in the region of the cleft.

Position of teeth. The lateral incisor on the affected side may be located in either portion of the alveolar bone adjacent to the cleft. The tooth or teeth will often be displaced palatally and rotated.

Eruption delay. There is often a delay in dental development on the cleft side, leading to delayed eruption times.

Occlusal effects

A Class III incisor relationship is frequently found with a centre-line shift to the cleft side. In bilateral cleft cases the deciduous dentition may initially be in Class I or Class II Division 1 arrangement, but by the early mixed dentition the effects of limited maxillary growth (see below) are often reflected in a reverse overjet. Unilateral cases will frequently demonstrate a crossbite in the buccal segment, especially on the cleft side, which becomes progressively worse anteriorly. There will usually be a gap in the dental arch in the line of the cleft as teeth cannot erupt or move into an area with limited bone.

Skeletal effects

There is often a Class III skeletal relationship, with both the maxilla and to some extent the mandible being retrusive. Until the age of 6–8 years the bilateral cleft has a protrusive premaxilla. However, with the restraint on growth imposed by the surgical repair early in life there may be change towards Class III (maxillary retrusion) in the early teenage years. There is also an increased anterior face height for both unilateral and bilateral clefts; a lateral open bite may also be found on the cleft side due to a localized failure of alveolar development.

Growth effects

There is strong circumstantial evidence to show that the surgical repair of the lip and palate early in life has a deleterious effect on growth of the facial skeleton, an effect that becomes particularly evident during the prepubertal growth spurt as a developing maxillary retrusion. This is supported by studies of individuals whose clefts have remained unrepaired. In Western countries it is unacceptable to leave a cleft unrepaired beyond the first year of life, and hence it seems almost inevitable that this compromise must be accepted. Currently there is much research interest in the process of wound healing, with the eventual possibility of manipulating the healing process to produce a scar-free result, with its obvious attendant benefits.

Hearing effects

The muscles of the soft palate act as a valve at the pharyngeal end of the Eustachian tube, equilibrating pressure between the middle ear and the oral cavity and allowing drainage of fluids. Repair of the soft palate cannot always ensure adequate muscle function. Despite early palate repair suppurative otitis media (glue-ear) is common. This will result in a variable degree of hearing loss, for

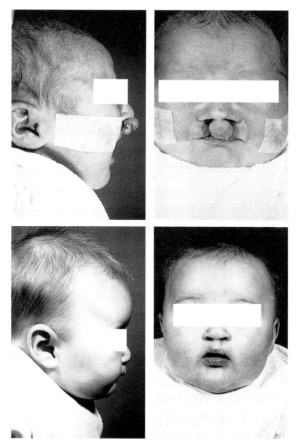

Figure 23.3 The same patient as in Figure 23.2 after three months presurgical orthopaedics. The lower pictures show the appearance immediately after lip closure. (Primary surgery performed by Mr M. Milling)

crossbite together with associated anterior displacement may be undertaken. This can be performed either with a removable or a simple fixed appliance. Care should be taken with orthodontic movement where teeth are close to the site of the cleft; in such situations, particularly if an incisor is rotated, it is only too easy to move a tooth out of alveolar bone with an inevitable consequence on the long-term prognosis of that tooth.

Later mixed dentition

Alternatively, and more commonly, correction of incisor crossbites may be delayed until the preparatory stage for autogenous alveolar bone grafting, which is usually performed at about 8–10 years of age. Preparation for such a graft may involve expansion of segments comprising the upper dental arch to achieve a normal form. A quad-helix appliance is often used to facilitate these movements (Figure 23.4; see also Chapter 17).

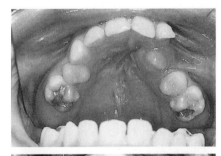

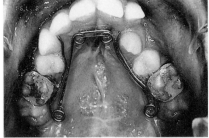

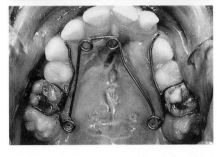

Figure 23.4 A quad-helix appliance being used to expand dental segments prior to secondary bone grafting of a unilateral alveolar cleft. (Records kindly supplied by Mr R. Samuels)

Shortly after the eruption of the upper lateral incisor and prior to the eruption of the upper permanent canine, if there is an alveolar defect, cancellous bone is grafted to eliminate the alveolar cleft. The bone is usually obtained from a donor site at the anterior iliac crest. The advantages of this grafting technique are that it stabilizes the maxillary segments, improves the vestibular appearance of the alveolar ridge, assists the closure of any fistula, and facilitates the eruption of the canine into the cleft site. Such treatment also facilitates orthodontic tooth movement and may allow a non-prosthetic rehabilitation of the patient.

Early permanent dentition

Extractions to reduce crowding may be performed at this time as part of a definitive orthodontic treatment plan; the initiation of treatment usually being delayed until the permanent canine has erupted through the graft site (occasionally because of local scar tissue this must be facilitated by means of an apically repositioned flap). Aims of treatment at this stage might include alignment, decrowding, dental centre-line correction and space closure or opening at the cleft site, depending on the case. Full occlusal correction in the early permanent dentition depends on there being no great underlying dental base discrepancy so that any camouflage necessary can be achieved by dento-alveolar movements alone (Figure 23.5).

The range of orthodontic problems presenting at this stage may vary greatly and therefore a dogmatic regime cannot be described; rather each case should be carefully examined and treated on its merits. Careful assessment will include an evaluation of the underlying skeletal pattern and the likely effect of any future growth. Where growth is adverse and the patient is developing a significant Class III incisor and skeletal pattern (with an associated poor facial profile), then fixed appliance treatment should be delayed to coincide with any planned orthognathic surgery.

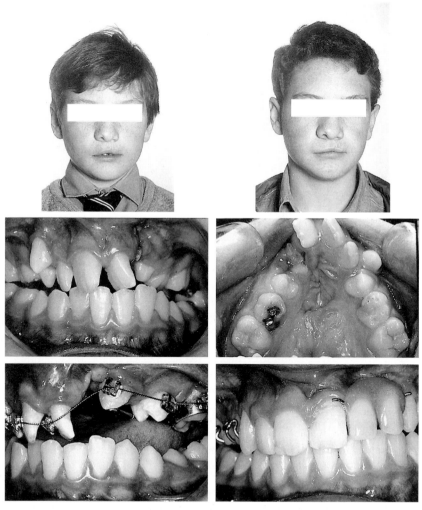

Figure 23.5 An example where correction of the occlusion has been by dento-alveolar movements alone. There has been a secondary bone graft prior to the fixed appliance being placed. A partial denture retainer is in place in the finish picture prior to a long-term restoration being placed. This would be either bridgework or dental implants. (Records kindly provided by Mr P. Durning)

Late permanent dentition (orthognathic surgery)

Once the patient presenting with cleft lip and palate (CLP) enters adulthood they should be reassessed. This provides an opportunity to examine the result of any previous treatments, which might include orthodontics, soft or hard tissue surgery, or speech therapy. Patients in whom large discrepancies of the jaws are developing may be identified. Many may have a significant Class III incisor and skeletal discrepancy with retrusive maxilla, such that the middle third of the face will appear flattened or 'dished in'. The patient's concerns, motivations for and expectations from treatment should be carefully explored at this stage.

As in all patients requiring orthognathic surgery, very careful planning is important with, in particular, maxillo-facial surgeons working closely with the orthodontist. However, other dental specialities may also need to be involved early in the planning process, for example, the restorative dentist may examine the need for any crown and bridgework as part of the overall plan for the occlusion and long-term stability.

The basic regime for orthognathic planning is very similar to that described in Chapter 22, as are the requirements for presurgical fixed appliance orthodontics.

Most frequently a maxillary advancement osteotomy, usually of the Le Fort 1 type (see Chapter 22), is an appropriate approach in these patients; very large advancements of up to 2.5 cm are sometimes indicated. It should be remembered that often the mandible may appear short in comparison to a normal profile (Figure 23.6) but it is doubtful whether mandibular advancement is often necessary. Occasionally, however, if a very large Class III jaw discrepancy is present a mandibular push back osteotomy as well as a maxillary advancement may be necessary to facilitate full correction of the skeletal and facial profile. In some patients movements of the chin (a genioplasty) may prove a valuable additional surgical procedure in improving the profile of the face. In the occasional CLP patient higher level Le Fort surgical procedures are appropriate. These will usually be at Le Fort 2 level, and sometimes in combination with Le Fort 1.

In contemporary management of CLP cases requiring orthognathic surgery the best results are obtained by moving the maxilla forwards in one piece following previous alveolar grafting (Figures 23.7 and 23.8). A careful evaluation of the cleft site should be made prior to the presurgical orthodontics, and where there is either a failed secondary graft (or more rarely none at all) the alveolus should be bone grafted at least six months prior to definitive jaw surgery. This later procedure is termed tertiary bone grafting.

Retention

Similar to other patients treated by these complex orthodontic and surgical techniques, in CLP all cases should have an individually prescribed system of retention and should be reviewed for a prolonged period of time. Whatever the method of treatment in CLP, stability is notoriously difficult to predict in these cases due largely to the variable nature of the scar tissue in the region of the repaired cleft; in many cases some form of long-term fixed retainer may be appropriate to hold expanded dental arches. One area where there has been good news in recent years relates to the stability of maxillary surgery in patients with repaired cleft lip and palate. If performed well, with good mobility of the upper

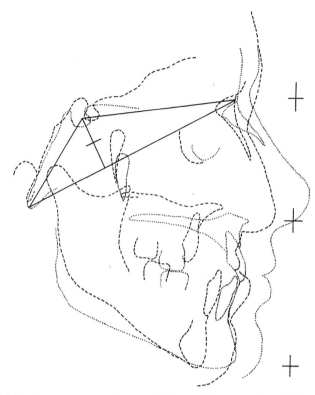

Figure 23.6 Tracing of pretreatment lateral cephalogram of the patient shown in Figure 23.8. This is superimposed on matched outline of a non-CLP patient

jaw being obtained prior to internal fixation, relapse of the horizontal position may be as little as 6.5% at one year post-surgery.

However, the vertical surgical correction remains a 'lottery', with an average of 16% change at one year (see Jones *et al.*, 2000). These results would indicate that orthognathic surgery performed well in cleft patients can show similar stability to non-cleft patients (13.5% horizontal and 33% vertical relapse at 1 year), at least in the medium term.

Some cleft patients on reaching maturity and when the above treatment is complete, will require late soft tissue revisions, rhinoplasty, pharyngoplasty and advanced restorative treatment such as fixed or removable prostheses or implant retained crowns. Throughout their first 20 years of life, the cleft patient will only derive the best from modern treatment if their dentition is maintained in good condition at all times. The role of the general dental practitioner in this is crucial.

Cleft lip and palate: centres for care

In recent years it has become widely accepted internationally that patients born with this condition are best managed, and that the most consistent high-quality

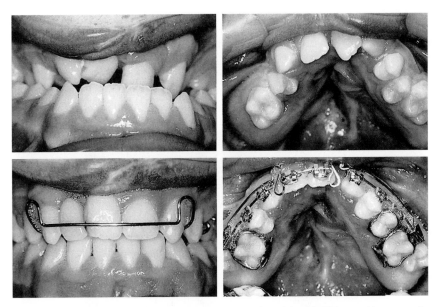

Figure 23.7 Pretreatment/post-treatment intra-oral views of an adult with CLP treated by means of fixed appliance orthodontics, an alveolar bone graft and a maxillary advancement. View on lower left shows occlusion prior to crown and bridgework but with retainer *in situ*. (The secondary surgery was performed by Mr A. Sugar)

results are achieved, in specialist centres. These should be of a limited number in any country and should have sufficient throughput of patients to allow valid comparisons of outcome to be made with other international units. In the UK in 1997 a report was published (see CSAG, 1997) which determined a national strategy of care. This followed an extensive nationwide audit of all 5- and 12-year-old patients born with a complete unilateral cleft of the lip and palate. This report recommended that patients should be managed in a small number of national centres with two primary cleft surgeons usually treating a minimum of 80–100 cases a year between them. Whilst it was thought important that surgery should be centralized it was accepted that orthodontics and speech therapy might be delivered on a 'hub and spoke' basis, with records, treatment supervision and audit being delivered from the centre. A similar approach has been successfully followed for a number of years in countries such as Norway, where there is a proven track record of consistent high-quality results (see Semb, 1988, 1991).

Other craniofacial syndromes

Of course cleft lip and palate is not the only condition which might affect dental and facial aesthetics and where a combined orthodontic and surgical approach may prove helpful. Other craniofacial syndromes (Treacher-Collins and craniofacial or hemifacial microsomia, Crouzon's, Apert's and Binder's syndromes) although all relatively rare, present on 'combined clinics' from time to time. It is

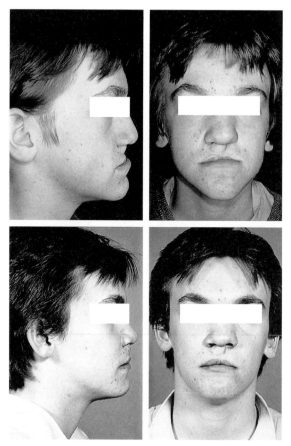

Figure 23.8 Pretreatment/post-treatment extra-oral views for the same patient as in Figures 23.6 and 23.7

not the place of this text to discuss these conditions in any detail. However, as an example of orthodontics and orthognathic surgery working in tandem in these conditions, the developing facial asymmetry associated with craniofacial or hemifacial microsomia can often be effectively intercepted early in the growth cycle by the combination of a costochondral graft and functional appliance. New treatments for this condition are also coming in to play in craniofacial centres whereby the deficient side of the mandible (and increasingly the maxilla) is lengthened by a process of distraction osteogenesis (see Chapter 22).

Conclusion

This text has, for the sake of brevity, concentrated on the orthodontic and maxillofacial surgical aspects of CLP treatment; it should be remembered that many other specialities are also involved including restorative and paediatric dentistry, plastic surgery, speech therapy, ENT surgery and audiology. All should form part of a co-ordinated team. However, in order for these children to obtain maximum benefit from the various treatment regimes described it is vital that both the parent(s) and child are dentally motivated from an early age and that a high standard of dental care is maintained.

Further reading

Boyne, P.J. and Sands, N.R. (1976). Combined orthodontic surgical management of residual alveolar and palatal clefts. *American Journal of Orthodontics*, **70**, 20–37.

CSAG (1997). *Clinical Standards Advisory Group. Report on Cleft Lip and Palate Care*. London: HMSO/Department of Health.

Habel, A., Sell, D. and Mars, M. (1996). Management of cleft lip and palate. *Archives of Disease in Childhood*, **74**, 360–6.

Jones, M.L. and Sugar, A. (1990). The late management of cleft lip and palate problems: a joint orthodontic/surgical approach. *Journal of the Royal College of Surgeons of Edinburgh*, **35**, 376–86.

Jones, M.L., Samuels, R., Sugar, A.S. and Newton, C. (1999). Outcome following maxillary surgery in cleft and non-cleft patients. *European Journal of Orthodontics* (Abstract 38) **21**, 443.

Kernahan, D.A. (1971). The Striped 'Y'. A symbolic classification for cleft lip and palate. *Journal of Plastic and Reconstructive Surgery*, **47**, 469–70.

Mars, M. and Houston, W.J.B. (1990). A preliminary study of facial growth and morphology in unoperated male unilateral cleft lip and palate subjects over 13 years of age. *Cleft Lip and Palate Journal*, **27**, 7–10.

Mars, M., Plint, D.A., Houston, W.J.B. *et al.* (1987). The GOSLON yardstick: a new system for assessing dental arch relationships in children with unilateral clefts of the lip and palate. *Cleft Palate Journal*, **24**, 314–22.

Nash, P. (1995). *Living with Disfigurement: Psychosocial Implications of Being Born with a Cleft Lip and Palate*. Aldershot: Ashgate Publishing.

Somerlad, B.C. (1994). Management of cleft lip and palate. *Current Paediatrics*, **4**, 189–95.

Semb, G. (1988). Effect of alveolar bone grafting on maxillary growth in unilateral cleft lip and palate patients. *Cleft Lip and Palate Journal*, **28**, 288–363.

Semb, G. (1991). A study of the facial growth of patients with unilateral cleft lip and palate treated by the Oslo team. *Cleft Lip and Palate Journal*, **28**, 1–21.

Shaw, W.C. *et al.* (1992). A six centre international study of treatment outcome in patients with cleft lip and palate. Parts 1–5. *Cleft Lip and Palate Journal*, **29**, 393–418.

Chapter 24

The orthodontic–restorative interface

This subject can be considered both from the standpoint of the contribution that restorative dentistry can make to the overall management of the orthodontic patient and also the role of adjunctive (supportive) orthodontic treatment in the solution of restorative problems.

The majority of orthodontic patients will be under the simultaneous care of the general dental practitioner, most of whom have considerable experience in restorative dentistry, and the orthodontic specialist. It is important that the complementary skills of each are employed to secure the most satisfactory and durable results of treatment. Inevitably this will involve consultation and collaboration during initial treatment planning and at all stages during the treatment. Occasionally, when an orthodontist is confronted by more complex and challenging problems, the involvement of restorative specialists will be particularly beneficial.

Restorative support to orthodontic treatments

The contribution of restorative dentistry to the management of orthodontic patients can be considered under a number of headings:

- general considerations
- alterations to tooth size, shape and colour
- endodontic treatment
- management of traumatic dental injuries.

General considerations

It is well recognized that proper restorative management of children during the development of the dentition can assist in preventing future orthodontic problems. Particularly important aspects are caries prevention and control. The provision of appropriate advice on the limitation of refined carbohydrates in the diet, use of topically applied fluorides and prescription of fluoride supplements are fundamental aspects in the management of all child patients, including those who may require orthodontic treatment at some stage.

Of equal importance is the management of carious lesions, should they develop, by appropriate restorative means. It is important that deciduous molars be conserved, by pulp treatment and stainless-steel crowns if necessary, so that they can fulfil the function of space maintenance for their permanent successors. First permanent molars also should be conserved. The loss of the first molar prior to the eruption of the second molar will make the use of space maintainers very difficult. Under these circumstances, the second molars, when they erupt, may be tilted mesially and rotated lingually. This will result in a less than ideal occlusal relationship with opposing teeth and may also complicate any subsequent appliance treatment. Should the loss of a first molar be inevitable, an orthodontic opinion should usually be sought by the restorative dentist concerning the advisability of balancing extractions of opposing and contralateral first molars also (see Chapter 8).

It is well recognized that placing any sort of appliance in the mouth, including fixed or removable orthodontic appliances, results in increased plaque retention in relation to the appliance. The restorative dentist must cooperate with the orthodontist in ensuring a high standard of oral hygiene in order to minimize the effects of plaque retention on the gingival tissues. This is important in the case of children, where the localized inflammatory response is likely to be reversible, but even more so in the case of adult patients, particularly those with an increased susceptibility to the effects of plaque, which may lead to the establishment or progression of periodontal disease.

Alteration of tooth size, shape and colour

The ability of the restorative dentist to alter tooth size, shape and colour by providing acid-etched retained composite additions, veneers and crowns can be very useful in optimizing the final result of orthodontic treatment, particularly in hypodontia cases (also termed partial anodontia). In these patients there may be a number of teeth absent, with those remaining of a reduced size. Occasionally teeth may be diminutive or conical in form (peg-shaped; see Chapter 8). The teeth most often missing from the permanent dentition are third molars, followed by upper lateral incisors, lower second premolars and upper second premolars.

In severe cases there may be a significant number of teeth missing (oligodontia). In these cases the early involvement of the restorative dentist in treatment planning to advise on the optimum final position of the few remaining standing teeth is vital. It is helpful to the orthodontist to have a clear idea of the likely prosthodontic plan before placing appliances. Treatment planning decisions may be helped by the use of study cast 'set-ups' as described in Chapter 21 (see Figure 21.2). They are particularly useful in explaining to the patient the likely outcomes of a variety of treatment options, and can be important in raising the patient's morale and securing their cooperation in what may be a prolonged treatment. Such an approach also forms an important part of the informed consent process in what are often complicated treatments.

In younger patients, where the upper lateral incisor is missing, a decision has to be made on whether to allow the upper canine tooth to erupt adjacent to the central incisor or whether to maintain space to facilitate later prosthetic replacement of the lateral incisor. The factors dictating this decision are discussed in Chapter 8. Whichever option is chosen, the restorative dentist has a role to play: either the shape of the canine tooth will require camouflaging or a prosthetic replacement will need to be provided.

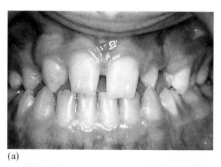

(a)

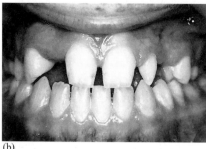

(b)

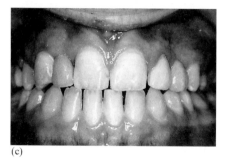

(c)

Figure 24.1 Joint orthodontic/restorative management of a hypodontia case. (a) Condition on presentation with missing upper lateral incisors (2/2), and upper centrals (1/1) malformed and the upper right permanent canine (/3) peg-shaped. (b) Completion of the orthodontic phase: upper right canine (3/) has been moved distally to create space for a prosthetic lateral incisor (2/); the diminutive upper left permanent canine (/3) has been moved into the lateral incisor position and a space is left for a prosthetic canine (/3). (c) Completion of the restorative phase: the residual median diastema has been eliminated by placement of porcelain veneers on the upper central incisors and the upper left canine (/3) has been veneered to simulate a lateral incisor. Saddles in the upper right lateral incisor and upper left canine regions have been restored by means of acid-etch/resin-retained bridges

Where the option of allowing the canine to erupt adjacent to the central incisor is chosen, the final cosmetic result may be compromised by the shape of the canine tooth on its eruption. On occasions it will be wider than the lateral incisor which it is replacing. In this situation the greater bucco-lingual width of the canine may dictate that it be placed in a relatively labial position so that it does not interfere with the occlusion. This may result in a square or flat contour to the dental arch of the upper labial segment.

Where the alternative option of regaining space to allow the prosthetic replacement of the lateral incisor is selected, the options are to provide:

- a removable partial denture
- a fixed bridge
- an osseointegrated implant retained crown.

Whichever option is selected it is important that the patient maintains a very high standard of plaque control. On occasions such an approach may be best deferred until the patient is of sufficient maturity to cooperate fully with the

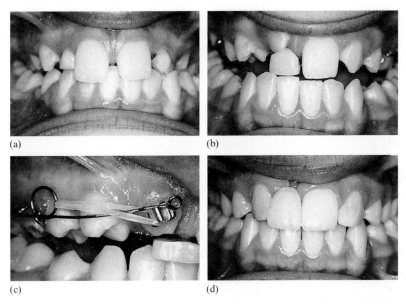

(a)

(b)

(c)

(d)

Figure 24.2 Management of a hypodontia case with missing upper laterals and an unerupted upper right permanent canine which has caused extensive resorption of the root of the central incisor on the same side. (a) Condition on presentation. There is a retained right deciduous lateral incisor with an attendant deep overbite and midline diastema. Note the tri-tubercular shape of the central incisors. (b) Following the extraction of the upper right central incisor the canine on that side has started to erupt. A temporary partial denture has been provided to improve the aesthetics. (c) Orthodontic phase. The right canine is being retracted to create space for a prosthetic lateral incisor. Some overbite reduction is also being undertaken. (d) Restorative phase. A resin-retained bridge replaces the upper lateral incisor and the shape of canine on that side has been modified by the addition of acid-etch retained composite material

maintenance of any fixed restorative work placed in the mouth. As a rule, implant retained crowns are the preferred long-term solution but age and/or economic factors may limit their use.

Occasionally the restorative dentist is called upon to give an opinion on the prognosis of standing hypoplastic teeth. One example of this may be a 'Turner's tooth', the permanent successor to an abscessed deciduous tooth; another might be a lateral incisor in the line of a cleft (see Chapter 23). Where extractions are planned these may be the teeth of choice; alternatively, if it is necessary to retain them, short-term options of composite repair or 'build-up' are available with the long-term option being a crown or veneer.

Endodontic treatment

Resorption of the root of an adjacent upper lateral incisor tooth may be one consequence of impeded eruption of a misplaced upper canine tooth. If the root damage is substantial it may be a clear indication for extraction. Alternatively, if an impacted canine has been surgically removed (see Chapter 20) any interruption to the blood supply to the pulp of the lateral incisor tooth may result in pulp necrosis. In these circumstances root canal treatment will be required if the lateral incisor is to be preserved.

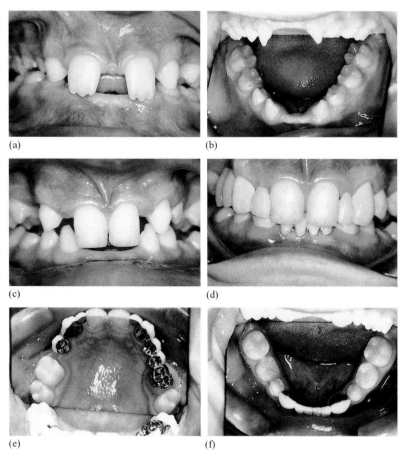

(a)   (b)

(c)   (d)

(e)   (f)

Figure 24.3 Management of a severe hypodontia case with retained deciduous teeth. (a, b) Condition on presentation. In the upper jaw there is a large median diastema, missing upper lateral incisors and only one premolar; the canines are malformed and there are two retained deciduous molars. In the lower jaw second premolars and all permanent incisors are absent, the canines are malformed and the first premolars are diminutive. Two deciduous molars are retained. (c) Completion of the orthodontic phase. The diastema has been eliminated and space collected for prosthetic replacement of upper lateral incisors and a second premolar. (d–f) Completion of the restorative phase. Upper central incisors have been modified by the addition of acid-etch retained composite material. Minimal preparation, adhesive retained metal-ceramic crowns have been constructed for 3/3. Bridge pontics replace (52/ 2)/(21/12). A first molar has had a metal onlay placed.

Management of traumatized teeth

It is important that any tooth tissue lost as a result of trauma is restored as soon as possible so that the full width of the crown is retained. If it is not, there may be a loss of space, which will then need to be regained as part of the orthodontic treatment so that the best cosmetic result can be achieved. This can be somewhat tedious for the orthodontist. In addition the condition of the pulp will need to be monitored so that prompt endodontic treatment, which may include apexogenesis or apexification procedures in the case of immature teeth, can be provided.

Orthodontics as an adjunct to restorative treatment

Orthodontic treatment for adult patients comprises as much as 50% of the patient load in many orthodontic clinics. Of these cases, many are adjunctive to support complex restorative treatment. It should be remembered that treatment times may be prolonged in the adult patient, they may be less ready to accept fixed appliances and be less tolerant of discomfort during treatment. However, there are a number of instances where such preliminary orthodontic treatment may greatly facilitate planned restorative treatment. These might include:

- teeth tilted, rotated or displaced buccally or palatally
- bodily repositioning teeth to permit optimum bridge design
- periodontally involved teeth
- rapid extrusion of teeth fractured subgingivally
- cases with deep overbites resulting in trauma to the palatal tissues
- patients with tooth surface loss.

Tilted, rotated or displaced teeth

In many cases, orthodontic uprighting of a tilted tooth, derotation of a rotated tooth or the alignment of a buccally or palatally displaced tooth may improve the prognosis for fixed, or less commonly removable, prosthodontic treatment. Subsequently there may be a tendency for the orthodontically repositioned tooth to relapse, and some form of prolonged retention may be necessary. This can present a challenging management problem. The involvement of the tooth in fixed bridgework will provide good permanent retention. In addition pericision, the surgical severing of the crestal periodontal fibres, may reduce the tendency to rotatory relapse.

Bodily repositioning teeth to permit optimum bridge design

When teeth are replaced using removable prostheses, these are not always effective in preventing movement of neighbouring teeth, which may ultimately result in space closure and a deterioration in the aesthetics with the development of occlusal abnormalities. Orthodontic repositioning followed by fixed bridgework may achieve a better long-term result.

Periodontally involved teeth

As a result of loss of attachment consequent upon chronic periodontal disease, teeth may drift and become cosmetically unacceptable. Provided that effective periodontal care is provided and that the patient maintains an exemplary standard of plaque control, orthodontic repositioning of the drifted teeth, followed by fixed retention, may enable the teeth to be preserved rather than extracted.

Rapid extrusion of teeth fractured subgingivally

Where, as a result of caries or traumatic loss of tooth substance, a projected crown margin is placed deeply subgingival, there is the possibility of localized periodontal problems as a result of plaque accumulation in relation to the margin. These problems are compounded by the difficulty in taking an adequate impression of the preparation margin. Rapid orthodontic extrusion, with or without repeated pericision, can permit the provision of a crown, which elicits a more favourable periodontal response. Simply extruding the remaining root will tend to 'drag' the gingival margin coronally as the tooth 'erupts'. Although a crown lengthening procedure would be possible eventually, if the discrepancy at gingival level is cosmetically unacceptable, an alternative is to divide the crestal periodontal fibres every 3–4 weeks whilst the extrusion is in progress.

Cases with deep overbites resulting in trauma to the palatal tissues

In cases with favourable skeletal and soft tissue patterns, it may be possible to depress the lower incisors, usually by using fully banded fixed appliances, sometimes supported by an upper bite plane. The result is produced by a combination of depressing the lower incisors and allowing overeruption of the posterior segments, both dependent on providing incisal contacts perpendicular to the long axes of the lower incisors for permanent stability. If there is an inadequate occlusal stop between the upper and lower incisors there will be a tendency for the lower incisors to be forced lingually, resulting in lower incisor imbrication.

Patients with tooth surface loss

As tooth tissue is lost from the occlusal surfaces of the posterior teeth, the palatal surfaces of the upper incisors or the incisal edges of the lower incisors, a number of mechanisms combine to maintain, at least partially, the occlusal vertical dimension. These include deposition of secondary cementum apically on the roots of the affected teeth and compensatory overgrowth of the alveolar process. The tooth surface loss is often confined to one part of the dental arch, usually the anterior sextants. Under these circumstances, it may not be possible to perform adequate occlusal reduction to accommodate a satisfactory restoration with an appropriate thickness of restorative material. In such a situation adjunctive orthodontics may be undertaken to create space by the method described earlier.

Further reading

Bishop, K., Priestley, D., Deans, R. and Joshi, R. (1997). The use of adhesive metal-ceramic restorations as an alternative to conventional crown and bridge materials. *British Dental Journal*, **182**, 101–6.

Evans, R.D. (1999). Orthodontic options. *British Dental Journal*, **186**, 605–8.

Oliver, R.G., Edmunds, D.H., Jagger, R.G. and Jagger, D.C. (1997). A combined orthodontic/restorative clinic. Rationale, evolution and experience. *British Journal of Orthodontics*, **24**, 159–62.

Chapter 25

Retention and post-treatment relapse

Relapse should be differentiated from the skeletal and dental movements that occur during continued dento-facial maturation. Relapse can be defined as the return, following correction, of the original features of a malocclusion. Unwanted tooth movements can result from periodontal elasticity, soft tissue pressures and skeletal changes.

Orthodontic stability demands appropriate treatment planning and a retention regime that prevents soft tissue forces and growth changes from disrupting arch alignment and interarch relationships.

Origins of relapse

Dental alignment is a primary objective of all orthodontic therapy. The dentition lies in a narrow zone of equilibrium between the resting pressures of labial/buccal and lingual soft tissues. Movement of teeth outside this area of equilibrium, by expanding arch dimensions or changing arch form, can result in a relapse, which is usually expressed as crowding.

In addition, when orthodontic tooth movement is complete, periodontal ligament (PDL) reorganization must occur to recover its original stable relationship. Within the alveolus, this relies heavily on osseous remodelling. However, the supracrestal gingival and trans-septal collagenous and elastic fibres have no osseous connection and often require some time to reorganize. These fibres have been reported to appear taut and directionally deviated after tooth movement, and the elastic fibres in particular can exert tooth-moving forces one year after appliance removal.

Finally, following the orthopaedic correction of skeletal discrepancy, a return to the original pattern of facial growth can be expected if treatment is discontinued before growth is complete. Similarly, a degree of skeletal relapse should be expected following orthognathic surgery. Both of these post-treatment skeletal changes must be considered when establishing treatment objectives and designing retention regimes to maintain three-dimensional interarch relationships.

Therefore, orthodontic stability requires appropriate treatment planning, an appreciation of post-treatment skeletal changes and the retention of dental alignment during periodontal remodelling.

Treatment planning

To ensure optimal stability of the orthodontic result, the transverse dimensions of the mandibular arch and the labiolingual position of the mandibular dentition should remain, largely, unaltered. Although the maintenance of the presenting lower incisor position gives no guarantee of absolute stability, the incidence of lower incisor crowding, post-retention, has been reported to be significantly lower when this strategy has been followed compared to cases in which arch dimensions have been increased.

A series of studies, originating in the University of Washington, have given an insight into the contribution of the orthodontic treatment plan to the stability of the result. These studies have focused on the incidence and severity of lower incisor crowding at the end of active treatment and retention. The treatment modalities evaluated included serial extractions (with or without appliance therapy), fixed appliance therapy involving premolar extractions and non-extraction expansion therapy. The majority of patients treated by each treatment modality presented with clinically unsatisfactory lower incisor irregularity when reviewed at 5 to 20 years after treatment. In all treatment groups – other than those where there was pretreatment spacing and those where mandibular incisors were extracted less than 30% of cases had satisfactory mandibular incisor alignment several years after treatment.

However, the changes in mandibular incisor alignment recorded in these studies have also been observed during the maturation of patients who had ideal alignment and interarch relationships without orthodontic treatment. In long-term studies, it has sometimes been difficult to differentiate between orthodontic relapse and tooth movements due to normal physiological change. Several authors have suggested that dental occlusion and alignment should be considered to be 'dynamic and constantly changing throughout the second to fourth decades' and, if dental alignment is to be maintained, permanent retention should be provided.

A final suggested contributor to loss of alignment following orthodontic treatment is the third molar tooth. If the eruption of this tooth generated a mesial force vector or if the presence of the third molar prevented 'distal settling' of the dentition during growth, then the third molar could be suggested to have a role in the development of post-treatment crowding. Conflicting reports have been published involving the study of patients who have congenitally absent or surgically removed third molars. In summary, if third molars do contribute to late incisor crowding, their role is a minor one and asymptomatic third molars should not be electively removed in an attempt to prevent late incisor crowding.

Methods of retention

The maintenance of interarch relationships and dental alignment at the end of active treatment demands a retention regime that considers postoperative skeletal changes and the forces generated from elastic periodontal ligament strains.

Where a presenting malocclusion was largely a product of skeletal growth pattern, continued postoperative growth could be expected to contribute to deterioration in occlusal relationships. Antero-posterior and, particularly,

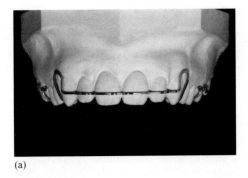

(a)

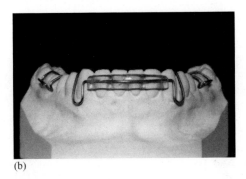

(b)

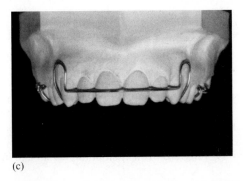

(c)

Figure 25.1 Examples of different types of retainers. (a) Upper removable 'Hawley type' retainer with fitted labial bow. This bow is formed in 'Edgewise' wire to hold incisor rotational corrections. (b) Lower removable 'spring Hawley' retainer. Standard removable retainer for lower arch. Note acrylic around lower labial bow to tightly hold alignment of lower incisors. (c) Conventional upper 'Hawley' retainer with a 'standard' labial bow from canine to canine. This would retain an overjet reduction with no prior rotational correction. (d) Upper removable 'wrap-round' retainer of the 'Begg' type. Labial bow runs from second molar to second molar. (e) Lower removable 'wrap-round' retainer similar to previous. (f) Clear acetate 'pull-down' removable retainer (made on heat/vacuum forming machine). (g) Fixed retainer for the lower incisors. This is made of stainless-steel braided wire fitted around the lingual surfaces of the lower anterior teeth. It is acid-etch retained to each tooth. (h) Conventional fixed lingual retainer for the lower labial incisors. This is acid-etch retained to lingual surfaces of lower canines only

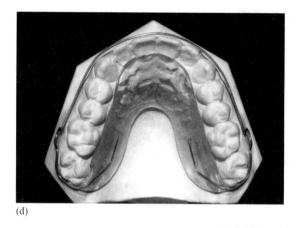

(d)

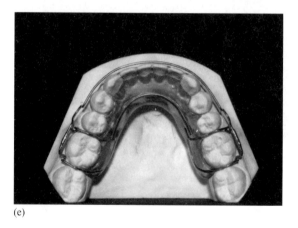

(e)

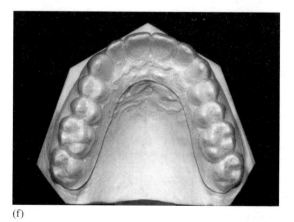

(f)

Figure 25.1 (*continued*)

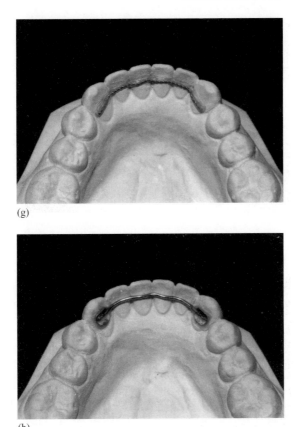

(g)

(h)

Figure 25.1 (*continued*)

vertical growth is commonly not complete until several years after active treatment is complete. Continued growth in the pattern that originally caused Class II, Class III, deep bites or open bites is a major cause of relapse. In such cases, 'active retention' has sometimes been advocated involving the use of extra-oral forces and functional appliances to maintain interarch relationships during continued antero-posterior and vertical growth.

The primary objective of an orthodontic retention regime is to maintain alignment during the immediate postoperative phase when the periodontium is remodelling. Histological studies have demonstrated that at the end of orthodontic treatment, the periodontal ligament will reorganize as soon as the teeth are free to respond individually to masticatory forces. This process occurs over a 3–4-month period. However, the collagenous gingival fibres reorganize more slowly, requiring 4–6 months, and the supracrestal elastic fibres can still exert tooth-moving forces at 1 year after appliance removal.

Retention regimes are commonly planned with this soft tissue reorganization in mind. For example, full-time retention is required for the first four months after fixed appliance removal. A removable appliance or non-rigid fixed retainer, that allows the teeth to respond to masticatory forces, should be used to promote periodontal ligament changes. The slow response of the gingival fibres demands that retention continues for at least one year. Removable retainers are commonly worn for 12–15 hours per day and, at the end of this period the elastic recoil of the periodontal tissues should no longer cause relapse. However, mindful of continued maturational changes, many orthodontists now advocate indefinite retention, using bonded retainers or removable appliances worn at night, to maintain dental alignment for as long as possible.

In an attempt to release tension and accelerate the return of the periodontal fibres to a passive orientation, 'circumferential supracrestal fiberotomy' has been advocated. This procedure (where a scalpel is used down the gingival crevice to cut the superior fibres of the PDL) has been demonstrated to improve the retention of incisor alignment post-treatment without compromising perio-dontal attachment.

Removable and bonded retainers

Removable retainers should maintain alignment and prevent the extraction space reopening following fixed appliance removal. They should not hold the teeth rigidly, allowing individual teeth to respond to masticatory forces, and should allow any favourable spontaneous tooth movements desired.

A large number of removable retainer designs are available, based on the base plate, labial bow and retentive elements of conventional removable appliances. The labial bow is designed to retain incisor alignment and can be constructed from round- or rectangular-section stainless-steel wire (Figures 25.1a, c). Where additional incisor control is required, the labial bow can be fitted to the labial contours of the incisors or can have acrylic added to offer the same control (Figure 25.1b).

Where elements of the removable retainer cross the occlusal plane, care must be taken to ensure that interarch relationships are not disrupted. To prevent occlusal interferences and allow vertical settling of the occlusion, a circumfer-ential design can be employed (Figure 25.1d). Alternatively, the labial bow can be soldered to the molar clasps to minimize anterior occlusal disruption. This design also is effective in holding extraction spaces closed (Figure 25.1e).

An alternative removable retainer design is the 'pressure formed retainer', which uses a 1–2 mm thick translucent acrylic to provide complete occlusal coverage (Figure 25.1f). These appliances are less bulky and, in the short term, more cost-effective than conventional retainers. However, they provide no facility for post-treatment occlusal settling and are insufficiently robust for long-term use.

Fixed retainers are commonly employed where the long-term retention of labial segment alignment is planned. They are commonly bonded to the lingual surfaces of the labial segments, either employing a robust stainless-steel bar retained by canine bonding pads or a section of multi-strand stainless-steel wire contoured and bonded to the lingual surface of each tooth to be retained (Figure 25.1g, h).

Bonded retainers are not without their disadvantages. Attachment failure can rapidly lead to loss of alignment, and plaque control around the retainer is demanding. Furthermore, responsibility for retainer maintenance should be established at the treatment planning stage. Therefore, careful patient selection is required before bonding.

In summary, a prescription for retention needs to be designed for an individual patient based on the original features of the malocclusion, the type of treatment provided and growth potential. A common regime, used to retain dental alignment, is to use removable retainers worn full time for 3–6 months, and for 12 hours per day for a further 6–8 months. Thereafter, the retaining appliances can be gradually withdrawn (two months night-time-only wear; two months alternate night-time wear) to assess the stability of the result. However, it should be noted that the retention plan should be tailored to the individual patient, and patients who have experienced significant orthopaedic changes during treatment often require more elaborate retention appliances to maintain interarch relationships during continued growth.

Methods of retention should be considered during the formulation of the original orthodontic treatment plan and the patient fully informed of the demands to be placed on them at the end of active treatment. Orthodontic relapse is commonly a product of the failure of a clinician or patient to understand what is required to achieve orthodontic stability.

Further reading

Blake, M. and Bibby, K. (1998). Retention and stability: A review of the literature. *American Journal of Orthodontics and Dentofacial Orthopedics*, **114**, 299–306.

An example of a standardized approach to orthodontic diagnosis and treatment planning

Assessment and treatment planning

1. Introduction and history
Age and sex.
Reason for attendance.
Previous illnesses and accidents.
Habits.
Assessment of interest and cooperation.

2. Soft tissue morphology and muscle behaviour patterns

Lips
(a) Morphology:
(i)   competent or incompetent;
(ii) habitual position – whether together or apart;
(iii) lip lines – upper, lower and active.
(b) Behaviour: the amount of circumoral contraction during speech, expressive behaviour and swallowing.

Tongue
(a) Size.
(b) Position – e.g. tongue resting forwards between the incisors against the lower lip.
(c) Swallowing behaviour – typical or atypical.

3. Skeletal relationships
Assessed clinically and verified from lateral skull radiographs if available.

4. Mandibular position and path of closure
(a) Mandibular position – rest or habit posture.
(b) Interocclusal clearance or freeway space.
(c) Path of closure – hinge movement from rest, or deviation or displacement.

5. Intra-oral examination
Clinical examination aided by models and radiographs.

(a) General condition of mouth

Teeth present:
(i)   erupted and unerupted;
(ii)   missing teeth (extracted/developmentally missing);
(iii) extra teeth (supernumerary/supplemental);
(iv)   ectopic teeth and pathological conditions (odontomes, cysts, etc.).

Oral hygiene – good, average or poor.

Periodontal condition.

Condition of teeth:
(i)   caries rate;
(ii)   damaged teeth/malformed teeth;
(iii) non-vital teeth discoloration, periapical involvement;
(iv)   resorption.

(b) Tooth positions and relationships
Upper and lower labial segments:

(i)   inclinations and rotations;
(ii) crowding/spacing;
(iii) relationship – midline; overbite, overjet.
      Upper and lower buccal segments:
(i)   inclinations and rotations;
(ii) crowding/spacing;
(iii) relationship – antero-posterior, lateral, vertical.

6. Diagnosis

Summary of salient features elicited in the case assessment (see 1–5 inclusive above).

Treatment plan

This is decided from the diagnosis, a stable final position for the teeth being all important. The cooperation of the patient and parents must also be taken into consideration. Treatment may be:

• ideal
• palliative.

Practical:
(a) General treatment – conservative, periodontal, etc.
(b) Orthodontic treatment – timing and expected duration, extractions, appliances, retention, prognosis.

A standard orthodontic diagnosis form

CASE SUMMARY AND PRESENTATION

This is .... He/she is ...... years old and is unhappy about ....
.... He/she was referred by .... who
was concerned about ....
He/she has been a regular attender at the practice for ...... years. He/she has a medical history of
....
Previous dental history of note: ....
There is *no previous/previous* history of orthodontics in the family. He/she is *unhappy/happy* to wear
a brace. Travel and/or time off work/school for appointments *is/is not* a difficulty. Other relevant
information ....

Clinical examination

The facial profile looks: *Class I*   *Class II*   *Class III*
with a *Normal/Increased/Reduced* anterior face height.   There *is/is not* a facial asymmetry.
The lips are *competent/incompetent/potentially competent*. There *is/is not* a tongue thrust on
swallowing.
He/she has/has not got a digit sucking habit. He/she has a Class .... incisor relationship.
The overjet is .... mm. on 1/ (mesial/incisal edge). The overbite is *Normal/Increased/*
Reduced/Anterior Open Bite and *incomplete/complete*. The dental centre lines are *coincident/not*
coincident. The upper centre-line is .... to the face. The lower centre line is
.... to the upper.
There *is/is not* a mandibular displacement from centric relation to habitual occlusion.

The displacement is:	*Anterior*	*Lateral to LEFT*	*Lateral to RIGHT*		
The oral hygiene is generally:		*Good*	*Moderate*	*Poor*	
The tooth quality is generally:		*Good*	*Moderate*	*Poor*	

The canine relationship is Class ...... on the LEFT   and Class ...... on the RIGHT
The molar relationship is Class ...... on the LEFT   and Class ...... on the RIGHT

The upper incisor teeth are:	*Crowded*	*Well aligned*	*Spaced*	*Rotated*	*Cross bite*
The upper LEFT buccal teeth are:	*Crowded*	*Well aligned*	*Spaced*	*Rotated*	*Cross bite*
The upper RIGHT buccal teeth are:	*Crowded*	*Well aligned*	*Spaced*	*Rotated*	*Cross bite*
The lower incisor teeth are:	*Crowded*	*Well aligned*	*Spaced*	*Rotated*	*Cross bite*
The lower LEFT buccal teeth are:	*Crowded*	*Well aligned*	*Spaced*	*Rotated*	
The lower RIGHT buccal teeth are:	*Crowded*	*Well aligned*	*Spaced*	*Rotated*	
The upper dental arch form is:	*Rounded*	*Tapered*	*Square*		
The lower dental arch form is:	*Rounded*	*Tapered*	*Square*		

Teeth erupted: _____/_____
Teeth restored: _____/_____
Teeth carious: _____/_____
Teeth of doubtful long-term prognosis: _____/_____
Other clinical features of relevance: ....

Radiographic examination

OPT

Unerupted teeth: _____/_____
Missing teeth: _____/_____
Displaced teeth: _____/_____
Additional teeth: _____/_____
Other pathology: ....

Lateral CEPH

SNA .... (Normal 80°–84°)
SNB .... (Normal 76°–80°)
ANB .... (Normal 2°–3° [Age/Sex])
Therefore antero-posterior skeletal pattern is: *Class I*   *Class II*   *Class III*
With *Maxillary/Mandibular EXCESS*   and/or   *Maxillary/Mandibular REDUCTION*
Maxillary/Mandibular Plane Angle .... (Normal (25°–30°)
Therefore vertical skeletal pattern is: *Normal*   *Increased*   *Reduced*
Upper Incisor to Maxillary Plane .... (Normal (108°–112°)
Therefore upper incisor is: *Normal*   *Proclined*   *Retroclined*
Lower Incisor to Mandibular Plane .... (Normal 89°–93°)
Therefore lower incisor is: *Normal*   *Proclined*   *Retroclined*
Lower Incisor to APo Line is: .... (Normal −1 mm to +1 mm)
Therefore lower incisor is: *Normal*   *Proclined*   *Retroclined*

Case summary

This patient has a Class .... Incisor Relationship on a Class .... Skeletal Base, with a
.... anterior face height. The upper incisors are ...., the lower incisors are
.... The dental arches are .... in the anterior +/− buccal segments. There
is .... associated with the cross bite. Additional local problems are: ....
....
Additional problems to be considered are: ....

IOTN   Dental health is ......   Aesthetic is ......

Recommended treatment

1. No treatment advised
2. Wait for further occlusal development
3. Extractions only
4. Tooth tipping with simple removable appliance   *+extractions*   *−extractions*
5. Release of mandibular growth potential using functional appliance
6. Three dimensional control of teeth using fixed appliances   *+extractions*   *−extractions*
7. Beyond the scope of orthodontics alone: *ortho/restorative*   *ortho/oral surgery*
8. Other solution: ....

Definitions

1. Soft tissues

Competent lips	A lip seal which is maintained with minimal muscular effort when the mandible is in the rest position.
Incompetent lips	When with the mandible in the rest position muscular effort is required to obtain a lip seal.
Anterior oral seal	A seal produced by contact between the lips or between the tongue and lower lip.
Posterior oral seal	A seal between the soft palate and dorsum of the tongue.

2. Teeth and occlusion

Dental arch	The curved contour of the dentition or of the residual ridge.
Occlusion	Any contact between teeth of opposing dental arches, usually referring to contact between the occlusal surfaces.
Ideal occlusion	A theoretical occlusion based on the morphology of the teeth.
Normal occlusion	An occlusion which satisfies the requirements of function and aesthetics but in which there are minor irregularities of individual teeth.
Malocclusion	An occlusion in which there is a malrelationship between the arches in any of the planes of space or in which there are anomalies in tooth position beyond the limits of normal.
Centric occlusion	A position of maximal intercuspation which is a position of centric relation.
Overjet	The relationship between upper and lower incisors in the horizontal plane.
Overbite	The overlap of the lower incisors by the upper incisors in the vertical plane.
Complete overbite	An overbite in which the lower incisors contact either the upper incisors or the palatal mucosa.

Incomplete overbite	An overbite in which the lower incisors contact neither the upper incisors nor the palatal mucosa.
Anterior open bite	The lower incisors are not overlapped in the vertical plane by the upper incisors and do not occlude with them.
Labial segments	The incisor teeth.
Buccal segments	The canine, premolar and molar teeth.
Cingulum plateau	The middle part of the palatal surface of the upper incisor.
Incisor inclination	An expression of the degree of tip in the labiopalatal plane.
Incisor angulation	An expression of the degree of tip in the mesiodistal plane.
Angle's classification	A classification of malocclusion based on the arch relationship in the antero-posterior axis.
Crossbite	A transverse discrepancy in arch relationship. The lower arch is wider than the upper so that the buccal cusps of the lower teeth occlude outside the buccal cusps of the corresponding upper teeth.
Scissors bite	A lingual crossbite of the lower teeth.
Leeway space	The excess space provided when the deciduous canine and molars are replaced by the permanent canine and premolars. The leeway space is slightly greater in the lower arch.
Primate spacing	A naturally occurring space in the deciduous dentition, mesial to the upper canine and distal to the lower canine.
Diastema	A natural spacing between teeth. A median diastema is found between the upper central incisors.
Dens in dente (dens invaginatus)	An enamel-lined invagination sometimes present on the palatal surface of the upper incisors.
Dilaceration	The deformed development of a tooth as a result of disturbance of the relationship between the uncalcified and already calcified portions of a developing tooth. Usually principally affects the root of an incisor.
Microdontia	Abnormally small teeth, often the last of the series.
Oligodontia	The developmental absence of a number of teeth (sometimes incorrectly termed – partial anodontia).
Odontome	An abnormal mass of calcified dental tissue.
Supernumerary teeth	Teeth in excess of the usual number – usually of abnormal form.
Supplemental teeth	Supernumerary teeth, resembling the teeth of the normal series.
Buccal segment classification	A classification of antero-posterior malrelationship according to the relationship of the mandibular buccal teeth to the maxillary buccal teeth. The molars are important in this classification but so are the canines (see Chapter 1).
Incisor classification	A classification of the antero-posterior incisor relationship. This is based on the relationship of the

lower incisor tip to the cingulum (middle third of the palatal surface) of the upper incisor.

3. Skeletal relationship, mandibular positions and paths of closure

Alveolar process	The parts of the maxilla and mandible the development and presence of which depend on the presence of the teeth.
Skeletal bases	The maxilla and mandible excluding the alveolar processes.
Skeletal pattern	The relationship between the mandible and maxilla in the antero-posterior axis.
Intermaxillary space	The space between the upper and lower skeletal bases when the mandible is in the rest position. It is occupied by the dento-alveolus.
Bimaxillary	Pertaining to both upper and lower jaws.
Prognathism	The projection of the jaws from beneath the cranial base.
Proclination	The labial tipping of incisor teeth often together with supporting dento-alveolus.
Positions of centric	The relationship between the mandible and maxilla when the condyles are in the retruded and unstrained position in the glenoid fossa.
Rest position	The position of the mandible in which the muscles acting on it show minimal activity. Essentially it is determined by the resting lengths of the muscles of mastication and it is a position of centric relation.
Habit posture	A postured position of the mandible habitually maintained either to facilitate the production of an anterior oral seal or for aesthetic reasons.
Interocclusal clearance	The space between the occlusal surfaces of the teeth when the mandible is in the rest position or a position of habitual posture.
Freeway space	The interocclusal clearance when the mandible is in the rest position.
Deviation of the mandible	A sagittal movement of the mandible during closure from a habit posture to a position of centric occlusion.
Displacement of the mandible	A sagittal or lateral displacement of the mandible as a result of a premature contact.
Premature contact	An occlusal contact which occurs during the centric path of closure of the mandible before maximal cuspal occlusion is reached. This may result in either displacement of the mandible or movement of the tooth, or both.

4. Cephalometric points and planes

Anterior nasal spine (ANS)	The tip of the anterior nasal spine.

Articulare (Ar)	The projection on a lateral skull radiograph of the posterior outline of the condylar process onto the inferior outline of the cranial base.
Glabella	The most prominent point over the frontal bone.
Gnathion (Gn)	The most anterior inferior point on the bony chin.
Gonion (Go)	The most posterior inferior point at the angle of the mandible.
Menton (Me)	The most inferior point on the bony chin.
Nasion (N)	The most anterior point on the fronto-nasal suture.
Orbitale (Or)	The lowest point on the bony margin of the orbit.
Pogonion (Pog)	The most anterior point on the bony chin.
Point A	The deepest point on the maxillary profile between anterior nasal spine and the alveolar crest.
Point B	The deepest point on the mandibular profile between the pogonion and the alveolar crest.
Porion (Po)	The uppermost point on the bony external acoustic meatus.
Posterior nasal spine (PNS)	The tip of the posterior nasal spine.
Sella (S)	The midpoint of the sella turcica.
Frankfort plane	The plane through the orbitale and porion. This is meant to approximate the horizontal plane when the head is in the free postural position, but this varies appreciably.
Mandibular plane	The plane through menton and which forms a tangent to the inferior border of the angle of the mandible (or alternatively through the gonion).
Maxillary plane	The plane through ANS and PNS.

5. Radiology terms

Kilovoltage (kV)	The potential difference between the anode and the cathode of an X-ray tube (in X-ray machine).
Milliampere (mA)	The current flow from the cathode to the anode, which regulates the intensity of radiation emitted by the X-ray tube (1 milliampere = 1/1000th of an ampere).
Relative biological effectiveness	A factor used to compare the biological effects of absorbed dosages for differing radiation and tissues.
Kilovoltage peak (kVp)	The peak value (in kilovolts) of the potential difference of a pulsating-potential generator.
Exposure factors	Radiographic kilovoltage, milliamperage, exposure time and source-to-film distance – all considered when making an exposure.
Tomography	A special technique which makes the image of a layer of structures more clear than those above and below.
Zonography	A tomographic technique which aims to see the whole of a structure in an undistorted and sharply defined form.
Cosmic rays	Radiation of extremely short wavelengths originating outside the earth's atmosphere.

Background radiation   Implies radioactivity arising from nature (e.g. cosmic rays).

X-ray   A type of electromagnetic radiation characterized by wavelengths of 100 angstroms or less.

Film speed   The amount of exposure to light or X-rays required to give image density. Film speed is progressively classified from A to F.

Localization   The taking of a film to identify a site in relation to surrounding structures.

Index